EHS Warrior

Beating Mold Illness, Lyme Disease, and Electromagnetic Hypersensitivity

Brian R. Humrich, Ph.D.

Copyright © 2020 Brian Humrich.

All rights reserved. No part of this publication may be reproduced, distributed, or transmitted in any form or by any means, including photocopying, recording, or other electronic or mechanical methods, without the prior written permission of the publisher, except in the case of brief quotations embodied in critical reviews and certain other noncommercial uses permitted by copyright law.

ISBN: 9798672040424

This book contains advice and information relating to health care. It is not intended to replace medical advice and it is recommended that you seek your physician's advice prior to starting any medical program or treatment. The author disclaims liability for any medical outcomes that may occur as a result of applying the methods suggested in this book.

Front cover image by Brian Humrich.
Book design by Brian Humrich.

First printing edition 2020.

www.EHSwarrior.com

To all the people out there suffering from Mold Illness, Lyme Disease, and Electromagnetic Hypersensitivity, **you are not alone.**

TABLE OF CONTENTS

Chapter 1- My Story	Page 8
Biological Treatment Center	Page 32
Natural Medicine Treatment Center	Page 33
New Results	Page 38
Detox Days	Page 40
Apheresis	Page 42
IRAD	Page 43
Ending Treatment	Page 46
Ketamine	Page 47
New Test Results	Page 48
Meeting Her	Page 50
Exosomes	Page 52
Tackling EHS	Page 52
Body Voltage	Page 54
EMF Challenges	Page 56
COVID-19	Page 58
EMF Free Community	Page 61
St. Johns	Page 66
New Supplements	Page 74
Sedona	Page 77
Conclusion	Page 82
Chapter 2 Connecting the Dots	Page 86
Chapter 3 Where I'm at Now	Page 98
My EHS Family	Page 106
Chapter 4 Weird Symptoms	Page 108
Inflammation	Page 109
Throat Problems	Page 110
Floaters	Page 111
Red Eyes	Page 113
White Spot	Page 114
Bleeding	Page 121
Hot-Colds	Page 125
My Penis	Page 134

Muscle Loss	Page 136
Emotions	Page 138
Sensitivity to Light	Page 140
Hair Loss	Page 141
Metal	Page 142
Tinnitus	Page 143
Pooling	Page 146
Episodes	Page 147
Weather	Page 151
Tile	Page 152
Heart Attacks	Page 156
Fingernails and Toenails	Page 160
Metallic Taste	Page 162
Inability to Sweat	Page 163
Random Rashes	Page 165
Detox Period	Page 167
Chapter 5 Other Things I've Tried	Page 173
Disulfiram	Page 174
Shower Filter	Page 177
Detox Baths	Page 179
Shielded Clothing	Page 180
Smart Meter Cover	Page 189
Driving	Page 194
Dirty Electricity Filters	Page 198
Floating	Page 202
Chiropractor	Page 204
Parasites	Page 206
VGCC's	Page 207
Dry Brushing	Page 208
Mold Candles	Page 209
Quitting Nicotine	Page 212
Earthing	Page 214
Rebounding	Page 217
Throwing out Everything	Page 218
Chapter 6 Threats to My Recovery	Page 221

Chapter 7 Basic Overview of EMFs	Page 226
Safety Standards	Page 230
Meters I Use	Page 234
Home Inspection Questionnaire	Page 238
Chapter 8 Supplements List	Page 242
Chapter 9 Further Reading	Page 244
Acknowledgements	Page 246
Contact the Author	Page 247
Other Books by the Author	Page 248

Chapter 1

My Story

My story does not have a beginning. The unfortunate reason is due to severe memory loss caused by my illness. Instead of a beginning, I will start off by introducing you to what I can remember.

I was driving when all of a sudden, my left shoulder began throbbing with pain. The pain shot from my shoulder, up my neck, and into my jaw. The pain was unusual to say the least. The only thing that seemed to alleviate the pain was applying constant pressure to my shoulder. Due to my history of injuries from weight lifting, I thought I possibly could have torn a muscle or pinched a nerve. The pain continued the rest of my drive home and long into the night. I couldn't sleep, eat or even concentrate due to the constant throbbing.

That night, I stayed up researching the muscles, ligaments, bones and whatever else I could possibly think of that could cause this sort of pain. I was healthy, in great shape, and had no clue what was wrong with me. The possibilities were endless in my opinion. I thought the worst and started creating a list of reasons I could be feeling this excruciating pain. The next morning the pain was gone but in its place was an uneasy feeling. What was that pain I was feeling? Was I imagining it? Was it all just a dream?

The thought of it being a dream began to sink in as I spent the next few days pain free. I felt off but chalked it up to my imagination getting the best of me. A few days later the pain came back but this time it was in my leg. It felt like I had a thousand bees buzzing around the inside of my leg, vibrating from the inside out. This was definitely not a dream. Once again, the fear of the unknown set in and I started to panic. I had no clue what was wrong with me. First, the pain was in one part of my body, now another? How is that even possible? What was the vibrating feeling? Am I dying? The pain was so intense that I couldn't sleep again that night and stayed up researching until the morning. That morning, the pain was gone but once again, the uneasy feeling remained.

That morning I remember feeling as if I had the flu and had the symptoms to match. I had an extremely high fever; I was throwing up nonstop and had severe diarrhea. That's where I thought I had figured out what the mysterious pains were. I thought that I was having body aches as part of the flu. My mind was finally at ease as I remained sick for the next week or so. Well, I was clearly wrong with my self diagnosis and that is where the "fun" began.

When the symptoms of the flu seemed to lessen, a new set of symptoms took its place. I had severe ringing in my ears, my jaw was sore to the touch and my neck was so stiff that I could barely turn from side to side. These new symptoms were like nothing I had ever felt before. My obsessive research to find out what it was, was inconclusive. Trying to explain the pain to other people left me feeling crazy so I kept the symptoms to myself. Looking back, that was a horrible idea. The pain soon made its way to my head, where simple tasks became increasingly difficult. Thinking became painful and talking left me out of breath.

At this point I was under the impression that what I had was rare and couldn't be found through researching online. My head constantly felt heavy with pain, my neck and spine were filled with shooting pains, my hands and arms were shaking constantly, my balance and coordination were completely off, I suddenly became sensitive to lights, and my mind couldn't process what was going on. I felt scared, alone, and a little crazy.

I don't really remember how I got to the point of putting tinfoil on myself to lessen the pain, but somehow, I got there. I had tinfoil in my shoes, under my hat, and all throughout my house. The craziest part about all of that, is that it actually lessened the pain! Although the pain was excruciating, I was at the point where I could do bits of research to figure out what was wrong with me. This is where I had figured out about Electromagnetic Frequencies and their effect on the human body. My symptoms were so similar to someone suffering from Electromagnetic

Hypersensitivity that I felt some relief when I thought I had figured it out. The relief was short lived due to the "inconclusive evidence" behind EMFs and their effects.

Once again, I stopped all research and began thinking this was all in my head and that I was just under a lot of stress. I took down all the tinfoil, and cleaned my entire house from top to bottom. My symptoms remained but I continued to tell myself this was just stress and to focus my mind on something else. I decided to go on a vacation in order to help alleviate the stress in my life and to my surprise, it helped. I spent the next week feeling progressively better day by day. The pain was now a subtle annoyance but at least it was bearable.

Upon returning home, the symptoms came back immediately. The shooting pain, numbness, tingling, vibrating and lack of breath were back and worse than ever. I felt like I was dying. Yet, I thought it was just the stress of being off of vacation and tried to ignore it. This went on for a few weeks until my body just couldn't take it anymore. I went to the doctors and tried explaining the symptoms only to be asked "are you hearing voices too?" They didn't believe the pain was physiological and thought I had a psychological problem. I left the doctors and headed back home, feeling crazy, but with determination to figure out what was wrong with me. If this were all in my head like the doctors suggested, what caused it to start? I was confused.

Some time passed and the symptoms seemed to get worse. I couldn't remember how to use my phone, I lost 55 pounds, multitasking became impossible, and basic words were easily forgotten. I reached out to my brother and he was extremely worried because I "sounded weird" over the phone. He contacted my parents and the three of them drove 3 hours to come and get me. They drove me back to my childhood home where I thought I was going to get better. That night I couldn't sleep and stayed up all night researching what was going on with me. I couldn't find anything other than Electromagnetic Hypersensitivity that made sense. My parents approached me that afternoon and told me that they wanted to take me somewhere. I asked where and their response was "you just have to give it a try", without answering my question.

Driving to the place where my parents intended to take me was far scarier than anything I could have imagined. They refused to answer any of my questions and wouldn't inform me of where they were taking me. In my head I thought the absolute worst. I believed they were taking me to a rehab center because they were under the impression that I was a drug addict. If that were the case, I thought that nobody there would believe me that I wasn't on drugs because I'm sure that's something others have said in the past. Then we arrived at a doctor's office, tucked away in a small strip mall of offices. Not knowing why they took me to a doctor's office, I remember saying under my breath "I want to run", which my dad replied "you better fucking not, besides you can't outrun a bullet".

I was absolutely terrified of what was going to happen as I stepped inside the doctor's office. There was a large waiting room, with children's toys everywhere, a large black sectional couch, and a humongous stuffed gorilla. After checking me in, my parents told me to sit down and wait. I continued asking why I was there and what it was for, but was ignored. Being treated that way as an adult was extremely disrespectful, and fueled my confusion and anger. Minutes passed and I was escorted back into the main doctor's office, which was even more intense than the waiting room. His office was filled with computers, lava lamps, waterfall features, neon lights, and numerous other technological devices. It was at that point that the confusion really sank in as I thought to myself "where the hell am I?"

After being bombarded with questions from the disrespectful "doctor" (I believe his disrespect came from his preconceived notions of what he was told by my parents), I finally pieced the reason why I was there together: my parents thought I had a drug problem and believed that neurotherapy would help.

Sitting in front of the doctor, they talked about me as if I wasn't in the room. Their words were hurtful and still hurt to this day. As I sat there, my left shoulder began to hurt to the point where if I wasn't applying pressure to it, I felt as if I were going to pass out. They did some tests on me, asked me a few questions and then hooked my head up to a machine. Their explanation of what was wrong with me was that my mind was stuck in "fight or flight" mode and they were going to reprogram it. None of this made sense to me but I went with it. After the first session I had an appetite again and felt a lot better. I scheduled a few more sessions and to my surprise I felt worse after each one but was told that "that's normal in the beginning". What did I get myself into? Why was I going to this doctor? After a week I felt like myself again and thanked my parents for helping me but I still had no clue what was wrong with me. I left their house with so many unanswered questions and returned to my house a few hours away.

My parents disagreed with me leaving their house but for reasons I won't get into. Let's just say they didn't like my living situation. The symptoms I was experiencing prior to treatment hadn't returned fully but I could feel them creeping up on me slowly. I knew something drastic had to be done so I completely changed my lifestyle in order to avoid being stressed out. This is solely because I thought stress was the reason as to why my symptoms were returning. I began meditating, practicing yoga, eating healthier, taking vitamins, and taking control of my stress. The symptoms stayed at a minimum but occasionally I would have "episodes" of extreme shooting pains that had no explanation because I was stress free. This is where my research began again. If it wasn't stress, then what was it?

I thought it could possibly be the house and returned to my parents' house once again. This time, things were a lot different. My parents were acting different and I had no clue why. My symptoms were worse than ever before and every time I tried to talk to them about the pain, it was dismissed and ignored. They didn't believe me and I didn't know why. I had no reason to make up these bizarre symptoms but whenever they came up, they were shot down with "the mind is a powerful thing". I can't even begin to explain to you how alone I truly felt. I was in pain with something I couldn't explain, and nobody believed me. I remember going upstairs, shaving, packing my belongings and walking out the door at my parents' house. If they didn't believe me, I didn't want to be around them.

My mom followed me outside crying and telling me to come inside so she could "get me help". I was confused as I got into my car and began to drive away, only to be stopped by the presence of my dad walking outside shouting my name. He stood there beside my mom, in his underwear, telling me that he "sees this shit every day" and told me to get inside. At that point the only thing that shot through my head was that they thought I was on drugs and my assumption was correct. My dad sent me a lengthy text message as I drove away telling me that I'm hurting my mother and to return home so I can get help. Here's the thing...I wasn't on drugs, but I was being treated like I was. Just as I thought things couldn't get any worse, I find out that my parents think I'm doing drugs and my brother thinks I'm schizophrenic. His explanation was that my symptoms apparently related to schizophrenia and therefore he assumed that's what was wrong with me.

Everyone in my family had their own opinions of me and what was wrong with me but nobody would listen to me. I knew this wasn't in my head but how was I going to prove that? And once I did figure it out, who was going to listen? A few weeks passed and I became extremely isolated with my symptoms. The doctors didn't listen to me, my family thought I was crazy and on drugs, and I still had no answers as to what was wrong with me. The symptoms got worse but I thought it was just because of the stress of everything I was going through so I stopped doing research and tried to convince myself that this was all in my head and that I had the power to make the symptoms go away. It didn't work.

I soon had nowhere to live, nowhere to go, and nobody to listen to me. So, I did what anyone in my situation would do, I turned to my parents again. The symptoms were so intense that I remember calling my mom crying and was told to "go to the emergency room". I felt scared to go back to the doctors because the first time I was made to feel crazy, but I went anyways. I left for the doctors and got so lost that it took me hours just to get there. By the time I arrived I was exhausted, hadn't eaten all day, and could barely speak. I walked up to the counter and said "I need to see a doctor; I think I've been exposed to non-ionized radiation." Through my research at the time I thought by saying that I could get the help I needed. I was wrong. Saying that made me sound even crazier than the first time I went to the doctors. They made me take a drug test and then sit right outside the psychiatric department. I talked to several doctors trying to explain why I thought I had been exposed to non-ionized radiation but the only words I could get out were "my hands..." before they would cut me off and tell me I was just under stress and that I was acting paranoid. Nobody, and I mean nobody, would listen to me. They told me they wanted to admit me but it was my choice so I turned around and walked out. I knew I wasn't crazy but they sure did make me feel that way.

Having nowhere to go, I slept in my car outside the gym that night. When I woke up, I went inside, took a shower and then returned back to my car. I didn't have money for food, a place to stay besides my car, or anyone that would listen to me. It was one of the worst moments of my life. I called my mom and asked if I could come home. It was as if I was admitting defeat and she knew it. I honestly couldn't take it anymore, and just wanted help. Everything seemed so foggy, and I questioned everything that I once held true to. As I drove to my parents' house the symptoms skyrocketed and my head felt like it was going to explode so I pulled over and turned my engine off. I remember sitting there with my head on the steering wheel, crying and asking myself why this was happening to me. I arrived at my parents' house that night and to my surprise it was even more uncomfortable than I had imagined. They truly believed I had a drug problem. After a few days arguing that I didn't have a drug problem I finally gave up and just did what they wanted in order to have a place to stay. I attended neurotherapy sessions daily, cleaned up after myself, helped my dad around the house during the day and spent the night crying due to the pain I was in from pushing so hard during the day. I made it my mission to figure out what had been wrong with me for so long while hiding the pain from my family.

After a few weeks I couldn't handle the pain anymore and went to the doctors again. This time it was a different doctor in a different city so I thought things would be different. I was wrong. The doctor wouldn't listen to me and told me that he wanted me to see a psychiatrist, so I did. The psychiatrist told me it was

PTSD and extreme stress due to a previous relationship. I knew that wasn't the case but I kept my mouth shut and just listened. I was prescribed an antidepressant and told to check back in a few weeks. I went home, told my parents and their response was "I knew it". That day I decided to take the antidepressant in order to please my parents and ended up feeling worse than before. I knew that I wasn't depressed, so I gave the pills to my mom and refused to take them again. My parents were extremely unhappy with that decision. After that, my isolation grew and so did my anger. I was angry that my symptoms still persisted and nobody would listen to me. However, I was still determined not to give up on figuring things out.

I researched everything I could (other than Electromagnetic Hypersensitivity) and came to the conclusion that I thought it was mold illness. It made the most sense and I found a naturopathic doctor that would meet with me. I couldn't drive myself due to my symptoms, so my mom took me to my first appointment. The doctor listened to me, which made me tear up because that was a first. She said all of my symptoms sounded like mold exposure but she wanted to do blood tests on me in order to be sure. Finally, everything that I had been saying (symptom wise) was validated and in front of my mom to say the least! What was even more reassuring, was that the doctor made comments on a possible link between mold and EMFs. I thought that for sure things would be different due to the validation. I was wrong.

The test results came back and they were just as the doctor had thought, mold. I was prescribed a protocol of medication to help detoxify my body from the mold exposure and was told not to start it until I was in a mold free environment. The thing is, my parents' house tested very high on a mold test but due to my parent's inability to "see the mold" they said the test was wrong. They truly did not believe that mold illness was something that existed, even with a doctor confirming that it did, or with test results to back it up. I started the treatment protocol anyways and started to feel a lot better the first week. After that first week, things got extremely worse. I was bleeding from my nose, my ears and throwing up blood as well. My body broke out into an incredibly painful rash and I felt like I had the flu all over again. Regardless of the new symptoms, I continued the treatment protocol until it's completion all while keeping my symptoms to myself.

After completing the treatment protocol, I did more blood work and met with the doctor again. The blood work showed the reason why I shouldn't have started the treatment protocol in a moldy environment. I got worse and this time I knew it was my fault. I now know that I shouldn't have started the mold protocol in a moldy environment. My doctor wasn't the happiest with my previous decision and therefore strictly stated that "if I were going to get better then a new mold protocol would have to start, and in a MOLD FREE environment." With that not being a choice, I took the new protocol and stashed it away for a day when I would be able to complete it in a mold free environment.

My research began again. For some reason, I continued to place my symptoms in various search engines, looking for other answers as to what was going on with me. I didn't believe it was just mold that was making me sick. After some time, I came across a disease that fit every single one of my symptoms...Lyme Disease. "There was no way that I could have Lyme Disease", was what I remember thinking while reading the description. However, something inside of me knew that I needed to be treated for Lyme Disease. I met with my doctor again and had asked if she could treat me for Lyme Disease. Her response shocked not only me, but my mom who was present. The doctor said it wasn't Lyme Disease and that it was just mold. She insisted that if we treated the mold, I would get better. She wasn't very nice about it though. Leaving that office, my gut still told me it was Lyme Disease so I leaned over and said to my mom "if I have Lyme Disease, I'm killing myself". This was said mainly because of the research I had conducted on what Lyme Disease is like. I knew that people who are diagnosed with Lyme Disease have two routes. Route one is that it is a mild or acute case, caught in the earliest stage, and can be treated with a course of antibiotics. Route two was the one I was scared of. It includes a long list of symptoms that continue to persist well after a course of antibiotics is taken. These individuals, from what I read, aren't living the best of lives. My mom looked over to me and didn't have to say a word, I knew she was concerned. If I had Lyme Disease, and couldn't receive treatment, things were only going to get worse.

At the next meeting with my doctor, my blood test revealed that I had some of the co infections associated with Lyme Disease. My doctor still didn't listen, and insisted that following the mold protocol was all that was needed. That was the last time I spoke with that doctor.

That next day I had a neurotherapy session that ended abruptly. Half way through the session, my mom received a phone call and stepped into the hallway. Seconds later she stormed in and shouted "WE NEED TO LEAVE NOW!! THE HOUSE IS ON FIRE!!!!" Stopping in the middle of a neurotherapy session was not advised, but my mom was my ride, so I had to leave. Little did I know, the house fire was my fault. I had accidentally left incents burning in my room and they had knocked over, causing my room to explode in flames. Our neighbor was the individual who called my mom and also was the first person into my house trying to put out the flames. The damage to my room wasn't as bad as the fear I had of my dad finding out it was my fault. So, my neighbor and mom agreed to tell my dad it was her fault.

After the fire incident happened, my stress levels were through the roof. At that point my symptoms once again took a turn for the worse. The Electromagnetic hypersensitivity symptoms seemed to pop back up and worse than ever. My life up until this battle, was filled with electronics, Bluetooth, and Wi-Fi. I had never even heard of Electromagnetic Frequencies (EMFs), or the affect they take on the human body. To say the least, I was unaware and unaffected. That quickly changed when my body began reacting to my cell phone and my computer. It was strange. My hands and arms would go numb within seconds of using one of these devices and then take minutes to regain feeling. With no logical explanation as to why this was occurring, I turned to the internet for answers.

My research methods were unusual. I would type my symptoms into the search bar and then click on the first link, lose feeling in my hands, read everything I could, wait for my hands to regain feeling, and repeat the process until I had my answer. From there I was able to determine why the tinfoil helped as well as why I felt the way I did when using various electronic devices. However, one question still remained: "Why is this happening to me?" Not only did I have mold illness, but numerous co infections associated with Lyme Disease and a sensitivity to electromagnetic frequencies? Three separate conditions that are all equally difficult to treat but also very similar in symptoms.

What was I going to do? I didn't have the option of making my home environment mold free because my parents didn't believe in mold illness, I couldn't get treated for the Lyme co infections because my doctor didn't think it was necessary (even though I did) and I couldn't walk around in tinfoil to protect myself from electromagnetic frequencies because that'd be crazy, right?

I'm not crazy; but wearing an outfit made of tinfoil would have certainly made me appear so. Instead, I found a way to conceal the tinfoil from others in order to avoid any confusion with my sanity. I applied tinfoil duct tape in my shoes, underwear, and underneath my hat. This seemed to keep the symptoms at a minimum but I knew it was only a temporary fix to my problem. I researched alternative materials that could be used in its place and discovered a fabric that was not only stronger, but looked less "crazy". The fabric was called "faraday cloth" and I immediately purchased some.

The numbness and tingling sensation that had spread from my hands and arms to the rest of my body was significantly reduced upon wrapping myself in the faraday cloth. I felt areas of my body regain feeling and a sort of "draining" sensation. After purchasing more faraday cloth, I fashioned a pair of underwear, lined the inside of my hat, and inside of my shoes. This method of protecting myself as well as alleviating the pain became my newest research obsession. I was able to find companies all over the world that produced articles of clothing made out of faraday cloth and began purchasing their products immediately. With each new article of clothing I wore, I felt my body regaining feeling in areas I didn't know were numb.

At one point I even asked my mom if she could turn the Wi-Fi off due to the research, I had conducted revealing that it was a major source of EMFs. Asking her that was met with a list of excuses as to why that couldn't be done, mainly because my dad didn't believe in EMFs or the damage they do to the human body. So, I took a cardboard box, wrapped it in tinfoil and created a shield for the Wi-Fi router. Whenever my dad was around though, it had to be removed because he thought that it was "crazy". Another method I tried was wrapping tinfoil around pieces of cardboard to place in my bedroom windows because there was a large high voltage powerline less than 50 feet away from the window. My dad noticed this one day, called me crazy, and made me take them down.

Any attempts made to get myself better by avoiding EMFs, wearing faraday cloth, or going to doctors' appointments, were never enough due to the environment at my parents' home. No matter what I did, I was still extremely sick but one thing was different this time around, I had answers. With nothing but my gut instinct to guide me, I was sure that I had Lyme Disease, Mold illness and Electromagnetic Hypersensitivity (EHS). The next thing I had to do was come up with a game plan for getting better, but that was nearly impossible with the brain fog, memory problems and overall sick feeling. Somehow, I worked up enough strength to pack my bags and head for a new state.

Prior to moving to an environment in which I could heal, my parents purchased their retirement home in Arizona. Once a month, my dad and I would drive 15 hours to the new home. Due to the fact that there was very little in the home, electronics wise, the EMFs were relatively low. But the drives themselves were brutal and on numerous occasions I felt like I wasn't going to make it. His car had Wi-Fi, he only stopped at fast food restaurants to eat, and talked the entire time about how much of a drug addict he thought I was. Those drives although brutal, taught me that some people are incapable of seeing anything other than what they want to see. It's never fun being called a drug addict when you aren't one, but keeping my mouth shut and nodding along with what he said was all that I could do, as I was trapped in a car with him.

I remember one trip in particular. Being sick with

parents who don't understand chronic illness is tough enough, but my dad took tough to a whole other level. He grew up in a "tough love" family and therefore empathy was not one of his strong suits.

We were out a restaurant with my aunt when the discussion of sleep came up. I'm not exactly sure what I said to my aunt but I believe I recommended turning off her Wi-Fi/phone at night. That simple statement sparked something in my dad who didn't believe in EHS or any of my other chronic illnesses. An argument ensued, leaving me more emotionally wrecked. He confirmed at that point more than he ever had, that he did not believe that I was sick, and that it was drugs and stress that was the cause of my condition. The truth was clearly not enough for him as he had assured in the past that it would be.

My dad was never the parent I went to with my problems, that was my mom. My dad was more of the disciplinary one. He was the one who unknowingly to him, shaped my ethics and morals into what they are today. Because of my dad, I don't lie. I learned at a young age that lying results in having to work for free on top of a roof in 100-degree weather. Remember that dad? I learned so many things from my dad, without him ever realizing he was teaching me. That's why him not being there for me was so hard in the beginning. He had always taught me that if I were honest, he would believe me first. That wasn't the case with my chronic illness. My symptoms were unusual and therefore, believing me wasn't the problem. It was him believing the symptoms that was the problem. The symptoms he saw reminded him of a drug addict, and being a police officer, he thought he knew what was wrong with me.

Not wanting to be alone, I had convinced my little brother to come with me. He had just gotten out of a long-term relationship, so in my head it made sense for him to come. We drove the next day to Arizona, a state in which I thought had less EMFs as well as a better chance at getting treated. We arrived in the middle of the summer, 118-degree heat, but I felt nothing. My bodies temperature regulator was broken and therefore I couldn't feel just how hot it was. Just for reference purposes my daily outfit consisted of full EMF protection insoles, socks, tights, underwear, two tank tops, two t shirts, two sweatshirts and special protection tape lining the inside of my hat. On top of all that was my normal outfit in order to hide everything from judging eyes. Nobody ever knew the extreme measures I took to protect myself from EMFs.

Why did I care about hiding my EMF protection clothing from the public? Simple, because mainstream media and doctors claim EMFs are not dangerous and individuals who wear such products are seen as "crazy". Like I said before, I'm not crazy, so why confuse people. It was just easier to not have to explain. Besides, wearing EMF protection clothing relieved a lot of physical discomfort, and I wouldn't have worn it if it didn't work.

The house we rented was small, had no carpet per my preference, and was miles away from the nearest town. It was in the middle of nowhere, perfect for healing. But healing was not what occurred. My brother being the avid gamer that he was, used Wi-Fi

24/7 to play his games, leaving me alone in my room to deal with the pain.

There was one benefit to being in this new home, it was completely mold free. Being in a mold free environment, I decided to start the mold protocol that I had stashed away. The protocol was strictly followed; for one month, I didn't leave the house, took my medicine, and kept to a healthy diet. The mold protocol, although followed perfectly, didn't work and left me thinking that a different approach was needed. I contacted a treatment center in Arizona that specialized in Lyme and Cancer and set up an in-person appointment, hoping that I was right about my condition being due to Lyme Disease. If that were the case, then treating it would "make me normal again."

The appointment was long and involved me telling my story up until this point. I mentioned mold illness and the protocols I followed as well as my belief that I had Electromagnetic Hypersensitivity (EHS), which was something he had never heard of so I avoided going into detail and finished up my explanation with my thoughts on Lyme Disease. The doctor asked me why I thought I had Lyme Disease and I told him the truth: "I just know". He claimed that while my symptoms seemed like Lyme Disease, he needed to be sure and asked if I could come back later in the day for some blood tests. Rather than driving back to my house over an hour a way, I sat in my car and waited for my appointment time. I was anxious to say the least. I had my blood tests done and then headed home to hear back from the doctor.

Days later I received a call from the treatment center. "Brian, hey, do you want to start your treatment now or wait for the results to come in?" Not wanting to wait for the results, I scheduled my start date with the treatment center. The next day I was instructed to go and get a perm-a-cath placed inside my chest in order to receive the treatment. A perm-a-cath is a device installed inside the right side of the chest that has two tubes sticking out, used to hook up into for direct IV antibiotics. My brother drove me to my appointment and waited in the waiting room in order to drive me back. This was because the surgery required certain medication that would prevent me from being able to drive afterwards. Getting that perm-a-cath in was the first step in getting treated for Lyme Disease.

The next day I woke up and drove an hour to the treatment center, by myself. It was one of the scariest/exciting moments of my life. My mind was filled with questions: what if I don't get better after this? What if I really am crazy and this is all in my head? How long will it take before I start seeing results? Rather than focus on the negative questions bouncing around in my head, I tried to stay positive. My first day at the treatment center went by extremely fast but for the most part, I remember it being positive.

The atmosphere was very calm and quiet. Walking in, you are greeted by name, and given a name badge with your picture on it. After that, you head down a hallway to a seating area where a nurse checks your weight, blood pressure, SpO2, and tells you which room you will be in for the day. The rooms were all relatively the same. They each had approximately 5-6 leather chairs in them for patients, and plastic chairs in between them for guests. I never had guests, so my chair was always empty. That sucked. A few nurses were assigned to each room and would be in charge of administering the proper medication to each patient. After sitting in an open chair, the assigned nurse greets you, checks your identification badge and then brings out your treatments for the day. Depending on the day, my treatments lasted in between 6-8 hours.

I remember being nervous whenever the nurse would attach a new treatment to my port. Not because of anything the nurse was doing, but because it was scary seeing two cords hanging out of my chest and being attached to an IV as if I were some sort of robot getting refueled. After each new treatment, I would sit there and think about what life would be like if I were a robot. Just kidding, I didn't think that. I actually would just sit there, all day, looking outside and wishing I were somewhere else and healthy. Periodically throughout the day, I would have nurses check in on me and ask about the overall process and if I were getting better. For the most part, I wasn't, but I kept hanging in thinking that one day I would just be better all of the sudden.

About a week into treatment, my Lyme Disease results came in and boy did I cry. The test results not only confirmed that I had Lyme Disease, but EVERY SINGLE co infection along with it. My doctor wanted to meet with me immediately and discuss the results, so I grabbed my IV pole and rolled down to his office. We talked for hours about everything I had been thinking up until that diagnosis. I was confused as to how I even got Lyme Disease. I hadn't remembered ever being bit by a tick, so how could I have gotten it? We covered it all that day but, in the end, concluded that there was no way for me to know when I contracted Lyme Disease but to focus on treating it now.

My doctor at this point, ordered a lot more tests and came up with a plan to get me healthy again. His opinion was that it was Lyme Disease and once treated, I would be able to regain my once healthy life. The plan he came up with was as follows:

Home Therapies: Coffee enemas 3-5x per week in the morning time.

Supplements: Biotics Nutriclear Plus 2 week 15-day detox.

Medications:

1. (Daily) Compounded methylene blue 50 mg
2. (Daily) Nystatin 500,000 units
3. (FRI-SUN) Dapsone 100 mg
4. (FRI-SUN) Alinia 500 mg

Procedures:

1. Oxy-Bosh 3x week for 8 weeks
2. NoZone with Argentyn 23 Silver pretreatment 3x week for 8 weeks
3. PEMF 3x week for 8 weeks
4. IVC protect 2x week for 8 weeks
5. Doxycline 2x week for 8 weeks
6. Rifampin 2x week for 8 weeks

7. Daptomycin (Non IRAD weeks) 4x week for 2 weeks
8. Daptomycin (IRAD weeks) 2x week for 6 weeks
9. IRAD 2x week for 6 weeks
10. Calcium EDTA 2x week for 6 weeks
11. MIC Injection 2x week for 8 weeks
12. MitoStart every Friday for 8 weeks
13. ALA every Friday for 8 weeks
14. PTC every Friday for 8 weeks
15. Glutathione bag every Friday for 8 weeks
16. PRO-NK every Friday for 8 weeks
17. Cyclodex 1x week for 8 weeks
18. Quercetin 1x week for 8 weeks
19. Lactated Ringer 1x week for 8 weeks
20. Apheresis 3x total during 8 weeks

Additional Treatments:

1. Biological Treatment center
    a. CryoFreeze Chamber
    b. Hypobaric Chamber
    c. Binaural Beats Therapy
2. Natural Medicine Treatment Center
    a. Colon Hydrotherapies
    b. Lymphatic Drainage Massage

His plan was thorough and was designed to treat my body for Lyme Disease as well as the co infections and help regain my health. At this point, I was extremely intimidated by what I was about to go through.

Biological Treatment Center

I don't really remember my first day at the biological center because of how early I had to be there. In order to still receive treatment at the treatment center, I had to go into the biological center first. Which meant I was leaving my house at 5:00am in order to make it there by 6:00am and start my first treatments of the day. At the center, my treatment started out in a cryofreeze chamber, which drops your body temperature extremely low and supposedly helps with blood circulation and cell health. All I ever felt was cold. Then, immediately after I would head into a hypobaric chamber for an hour. This device was supposed to replicate high and low altitude training and help with oxygen flow. In the chamber I only ever felt stuffed and my ears would constantly pop. After that, I would then head to a third room, get hooked up to a binaural beats' headset, probes attached to my throat, oxygen attached to my nose and fall asleep for thirty minutes. This was supposed to retrain my brain as well as recharge it. All I can tell you about that is that I remember taking amazing naps.

After two hours at the biological center, I would head to the treatment center where I would receive IV treatments for 6-8 hours. However, my days didn't always end there. Once a week I also had to receive colon hydrotherapies, and lymphatic drainage massage. Those days literally "sucked". At this point, my days were endless, and my symptoms weren't getting any better. My doctors continued to assure me that I was going to feel worse before I felt better. Hearing that helped, but didn't make my symptoms go away.

BRIAN R. HUMRICH

Natural Medicine Treatment Center

The other treatment center I was instructed to go to by my doctor was a "Natural Medicine Treatment Center". For reasons not explained, I was told to go there once a week for 8 weeks and receive additional treatments.

At first, I despised going there. It was confusing getting there, even though it was only 5 minutes away from my main treatment center. But having brain fog and difficulties with my memory meant that even the easiest tasks were now difficult.

Entering the natural treatment center, you first walk into a waiting room area with a large flat screen television, a few chairs, and are greeted by a receptionist sitting behind a large desk with two computers. On a large chalkboard behind the receptionist is the quote:

"The doctor of the future will give no medication but will interest their patients in the care of the human frame, diet, and in the cause and prevention of disease"- Thomas Edison.

After getting checked in, you are then walked back to the treatment area where your first treatment begins. Not knowing what my treatments were I was scared, but the doctor performing my first treatment was nice and gave me a rundown prior to beginning.

The first treatment was a "lymphatic drainage massage". Sounds simple enough, right? Wrong. The treatment was not a massage. It was 45 minutes of torture. Let me explain why it was torturous. The doctor first had me get undressed in a private room (everything but my underwear), which made me uncomfortable because that meant taking off my EMF protection clothing. Then I was instructed to lie down on a massage table face up, with a sheet and towel covering the lower half of my body. After that, the doctor came into the room, turned on a large device behind my head and pulled out two large glass wands. The wands were attached to the large machine and a current of electricity surged into them, creating a static electricity field.

If that wasn't scary enough, the doctor then proceeded to rub the electricity filled wands down my body, attempting to drain my lymphatic system. Normally that wouldn't be that big of a deal, but being electrically sensitive made it painful. The entire time the "massage" was going on, I felt my body melting into the table. The melting sensation was something I was familiar with as it was a common symptom I experienced around high levels of EMFs. It was an extremely surreal experience that activated each of my symptoms and therefore resulted in me feeling tortured. Afterwards, I was instructed to come back the next day for another treatment, a colon hydrotherapy.

The next day I arrived at the natural treatment center extremely tired. The night before I didn't sleep for two reasons- 1. My EHS symptoms were flaring up (possibly from the lymphatic drainage massage) and 2. Because I was scared of getting a colon hydrotherapy.

My first colon hydrotherapy was with a different individual than I had the previous day. She wasn't a doctor but was a specialist, to be specific she was a "colon hydrotherapist". After checking in, she walked me back to a room I hadn't been in before and handed me a medical robe (the ones that open in the back) and a towel, and told me to change into it, lay down on the table, and press a Bluetooth enabled button that would inform her I was ready to begin.

The room itself was very intimidating. It had a single exam/massage table, a toilet in the corner with a curtain covering it, a chair for my belongings, a swivel chair for the specialist, a small table with an ungrounded lamp (I checked), an Alexa enabled device, and a large machine with tubes coming out of it in another corner.

After changing into the medical robe and pressing the Bluetooth enabled button, the specialist came in the room and had me lay on my left side revealing my buttocks. At that point she lubricated a large plastic tube called a speculum, inserted into my anus, and had me roll back over, slowly, onto my back. That was by far the worst part. Don't laugh, I'm a baby. Water was then sprayed into my colon, something she called a "fill". With each fill, the goal was to hold as much water inside of me. Since there was no unit of measurement as to how much water I was holding, time was used. Typically, I could handle approximately 30 seconds to a minute worth of water. After each fill, the speculum would then suck the water back out, in an attempt to get out everything inside the colon. Along with the speculum sucking, the specialist would rub my stomach from side to side, helping the water and anything else in my colon make its way out of me. I thought of this process as "assisted pooping".

The whole process lasted about an hour, going back and forth from filling to sucking. Due to the fact that my doctor never explained why he prescribed these treatments; my understanding was because of my toxicity level as well as my inability to detox on my own. The colon hydrotherapies assisted my body in detoxing what I naturally was unable to because of my condition.

Over the next few weeks/treatments at the Natural Medicine Treatment center, I worked up enough courage to finally mention to the doctor that the lymphatic drainage massage was making me worse. After discussing that I was EHS, the doctor shouted "WHY DIDN'T YOU TELL ME?!" Electromagnetic sensitivities were something she was familiar with and therefore knew why I was feeling worse with each treatment. After that, she no longer used the electrical wands on me and instead used her hands to drain my lymphatic system. That is when I switched from my original disposition of despising the place, to actually enjoying and looking forward to each treatment.

Months later with the permission of the doctor, I brought my EMF meters into the treatment center and showed her what I was experiencing while the wands were on my body. With my body voltage meter in hand, and the wands touching my body, my body voltage was well over 2,000 millivolts. That alone astonished the doctor to the point of making her EMF proof her entire office.

She got rid of her Alexa device, which had readings in the thousands even when switched off. She grounded her lamp in the colon hydrotherapy room, which was creating excess dirty electricity. She grounded the desk in her office, which was causing her body voltage to exceed safe limits (800 millivolts prior to grounding, 45 millivolts after). She got rid of all her Bluetooth enabled devices like her keyboard and mouse, which were putting off spikes of radio frequencies so high that the meters I had couldn't read them. She disconnected the large flat screen television in the waiting room, which was a "smart television" and putting off extremely high levels of radio frequencies even while it was off. She purchased dirty electricity filters which lowered her dirty electricity levels from 300 millivolts to under 50 millivolts. She even got rid of Wi-Fi and wired her entire office space with Ethernet connectivity. If that weren't enough, she also began carrying blue light blocking glasses for patients. Everything that I suggested, she did. Not for me, but because she saw first-hand the benefit of a reduced EMF lifestyle.

Now, the only issue with the natural treatment center is the radio frequencies coming from the Wi-Fi routers of the adjoining suites. Something that can only be fixed by using radio frequency shielding paint or by having the adjoining suites switch to an Ethernet based internet option rather than Wi-Fi. Still, she was able to reduce the overall EMFs in her office by 90% and has benefited tremendously.

Looking back, I wish I would have said something

sooner about me being EHS but at least moving forward I don't have to worry as much when I am in that office.

New Results

At home, I was trying to keep up with the new diet assigned to me. I say assigned, because I wasn't given a choice. If I wanted to get better, I had to be strict in everything. My diet was the keto diet. High fat, high protein, low carb, no sugar, no dairy, basically. Sticking to that diet was easy, mainly because I never had an appetite. A typical daily meal schedule looked like this: breakfast would be either two eggs with bacon or nothing depending on the day. Half the week I had to "fast" before my first treatment so breakfast wasn't an option. Lunch was always eaten at the treatment center and consisted of strawberries, nuts, a gluten free/dairy free sandwich, and a protein shake. Dinner was typically the same as lunch or nothing at all. My diet was boring but at least I knew exactly what was going into my body. Or so I thought.

Weeks later I remember getting called into my doctor's office while at the treatment center to discuss the latest test results. Every one of my gut instincts was correct. I not only had Lyme Disease along with all of its co infections, but extremely high levels of mold in my body as well as numerous other environmental toxins. Although the results were shocking to the doctor, I remember feeling happy. Happy because I was right all along and now, I had a mountain of proof as to why. The results provided by the doctor were as follows:

Lyme Disease (the numbers represent the infection load count at the time of the test)

1. Anaplasma phagocytophilium- 8
2. Babesia divergens- 126
3. Babesia microti- 26
4. Bartonella bacilliformis - 7
5. Bartonella henselae - 37
6. Bartonella Quintana - 38
7. Borrelia burgdorferi – 145
8. Borrelia miyamotoi - 47
9. Borrelia recurrentis - 9
10. Ehrlichia chaffeensis - 123
11. Rickettsia rickettsia - 21
12. Chryseobacterium species - 133
13. Staphylococcus haemolyticus - 159
14. Staphylococcus lugdunensis – 6,458
15. Streptococcus anginosus – 8,840
16. Streptococus intermedius – 13,904
17. Streptococcus urinalis – 41,766
18. Veillonella atypica - 423

Mold

1. Aflatoxin-M1 (Aspergillus)- 3.50 ng/g, safe reference range is < 3.5
2. Ochratoxin A (Aspergillus) – 11.41 ng/g, safe reference range is < 4
3. Mycophenolic Acid (Penicillum) – 255.84 ng/g, safe reference range is < 5
4. Verrucarin A (Stachybotrys) – 5.25 ng/g, safe reference range is < 1
5. Chaetoglobosin A (Chaetomium globosum) – 67.19 ng/g, safe reference range is < 20

Environmental Toxins

1. 2-Hydroxyisobutyric acid (2HIB) – 13,635 µg/g, safe reference range is < 200
2. Monoethylphthalate (MEP) – 162 µg/g, safe reference range is < 5
3. 2-3-4 Methylhippuric Acid (2,-3,4-MHA) – 286 µg/g, safe reference range is < 10
4. Phenylglyoxylic Acid (PGO) – 602 µg/g, safe reference range is < 5
5. Perchlorate (PERC) – 25 µg/g, safe reference range is < 2
6. N-acetyl(2-hydroxypropyl)cysteine (NAHP) - 98 µg/g, safe reference range is < 4
7. N-acetyl-S-(2-carbamoylethyl)cysteine (NAE) – 124 µg/g, safe reference range is < 4
8. N-acetyl(3,4-dihydroxybutyl)cysteine (NADB) - 227 µg/g, safe reference range is < 4
9. Tiglylglycine (TG) – 2.4 mmol/mol, safe reference range is < .04

The next day my treatment protocols changed slightly in order to combat the additional toxin load in my body. I started to get better and finally started to see myself getting better. I was following my doctors' protocol exactly how it was advised.

Detox Days

Fridays were the longest day of treatments and consisted of mainly detox protocols. After two hours at the biological treatment center, Friday detox day would begin at the Lyme and Cancer treatment center. All together Fridays consisted of approximately 12 hours of treatments, and were amongst the more beneficial days. Out of all of the Friday treatments, two stood out the most for me: Mitostart, and Glutathione.

Mitostart was a treatment that was designed to treat my mitochondrion health. It had to be attached to a machine on my IV pole where its drip rate was monitored closely. This was by far the most intense IV treatment, as it made me pass out on numerous occasions and always made my heart beat erratically. Talking with my doctor about how Mitostart made me feel, he made suggestions to the nurses assigned to me that would prevent me from passing out. After making his recommendations, I typically would only feel dizzy, nauseous, or my heart would beat erratically; and the passing out stopped.

After receiving the Mitostart treatment, I then went through my next several treatments with ease. For approximately 7 more hours, I would sit by myself and receive treatment after treatment. Then towards the end of the day, and being one of the only individuals left, I received my final treatment, Glutathione. Depending on how late it was in the day, I would either receive a direct injection into the tubes coming out of my chest, or be hooked up to an additional IV pole. If it was injected into my chest, it took around 1 minute to complete the treatment and was called a "Glutathione push". I preferred the IV version, as it took approximately 1 hour to slowly enter my body and seemed more beneficial in my opinion.

Leaving the treatment center on Fridays, I would feel better than I had all week. My symptoms were still there, but something inside me knew that Friday detox days were actually doing something. The reason why they were called detox days was because the treatments were geared towards detoxing my body from the inside out. Getting home on Fridays, I would then take a detox bath and attempt to go to sleep, but would usually lay awake in bed staring at the green smoke detector light until the effects of the treatment wore off and I passed out from the pain of my symptoms.

Apheresis

One of the most intense treatments I remember was apheresis. This was where my port was hooked up to a large machine that cycled my blood out, cleaned it, and put it back in. The nurses in that room were amazing and made me feel extremely comfortable. Knowing about my Electromagnetic hypersensitivity as well as my sensitivity to lights, they would shut the lights off prior to me entering the room. The end of the treatment was somewhat of a group event, where nurses would gather in the room in hopes to see the "jellyfish".

Jellyfish is what the nurses called the biofilms found in the bag attached to the machine after apheresis. As the blood comes out of the body and is cleaned, biofilms are left inside a yellow liquid bag. At the end of each treatment, you get a chance to see just how well the machine worked by seeing what was floating in your bag. The first time I ever had this done, the nurse looked over at me with her mouth wide open and said "I've never seen one this big!" My jellyfish were huge and took up a majority of the bag. I remember wondering if this was good or bad and even asked the nurse. Her response was "well, would you rather have that in you still?" I liked her response because no, I didn't want it in me still.

IRAD

Every Tuesday and Thursday while attending the Lyme and Cancer treatment center, I had a treatment called "IRAD". These treatment days were among my least favorite due to the poor set up of the actual room, the close proximity of other patients, and most of all because of the intensity of the treatment itself.

The IRAD treatment was conducted in a room separate from the other treatment rooms. The room had two separate entrances, one of which was always blocked by the guests of the other patients. Walking into the only available entrance, you are immediately stared at by all of the patients and guests that are jam packed within the room. To the left of the entrance was two patient chairs, and three guest chairs. Across from the chairs was the staff desk where the nurses tracked each patient as well as prepared the medicine for treatment. To the right of the entrance was five more patient chairs as well as guest chairs in between them. At any given time, the IRAD room contained the most patients, guests, and staff, with an average combined total of 17 people.

The day before an IRAD treatment, you are told by your nurse not to consume any food for a minimum of 8 hours prior to the start of treatment. You are also told to bring a lunch consisting of fruits and proteins.

The next day, once inside the room and sitting in a patient chair, a nurse comes over and greets you by name and asks you when the last time you consumed food was as well as checks your weight, asks your height, and checks your blood pressure. After all the initial checks are completed, you are then administered the first treatment of the day. The first treatment was typically a round of IV antibiotics and lasted for approximately 1 hour. After that treatment is completed, a nurse comes over, pricks your finger and tests your blood sugar in order to establish a baseline starting point. Then an additional treatment is administered to drop your blood sugar. That treatment lasted approximately 45 minutes and blood sugar levels were then retested. Once the levels were low enough, the actual IRAD treatment was administered.

The reason why my blood sugar had to drop to a very low level was because then the blood brain barrier would open up, allowing the IRAD treatment to reach my brain. Apparently, from what I was told, Lyme disease was capable of getting through the blood brain barrier, whereas antibiotics are not. Therefore, by opening the blood brain barrier through lowering blood sugar with a specific medication, the antibiotics are then able to reach the brain for treatment.

When my blood sugar was low enough and the IRAD treatment began, I felt very dizzy and had a euphoric feeling surging through my body. The nurse assigned to me that day would check on me every minute during that treatment and would check my blood sugar levels periodically to make sure it wasn't dropping to an unsafe level. After completing the

IRAD treatment, you are then told to begin eating the lunch you brought. While eating you are hooked up to an additional treatment bag that is intended to help bring your blood sugar levels back up and close up the blood brain barrier. That part was always easy for me, since the food tasted amazing after not eating for a prolonged period of time and having such low blood sugar.

The part that was difficult for me was the actual dropping of my blood sugar. While my blood sugar was low and feeling the dizziness set in, guests of the other patients in the room always wanted to talk to me. They would ask what I was there for, why I didn't have guests of my own, and worst of all they would be on their cell phones or personal laptops. Being EHS, I could barely stand the constant bombardment of EMFs in such a close proximity and usually just pretended I was asleep in order to avoid people talking to me.

After that, additional treatments were administered within the room. However, on some occasions I was moved to a separate room due to poor planning on their part and having too many individuals scheduled for IRAD that day. I was typically one of the only individuals present in the "overflow" room and would finish out my final treatments for the day alone. There was one nurse though that would periodically check in on me and talk to me about life, she was remarkable at her job and made IRAD days more tolerable.

Ending Treatment

Half way through my treatment process, my brother left me alone in Arizona. He wasn't happy in Arizona and decided to move back. It was hard enough being in a new state, but now I was alone. Up until this point, I had at least felt minimal support from one of my family members, my brother and after he left, we stopped speaking. Now I was alone and had nothing of a support system to rely on for help. Not that I ever did.

Being sensitive to EMFs contributed to my loneliness. If I were ever lonely in the past, I could pick up my phone and make a call or send a text message. I could even flip the television on and zone out watching movies to distract my mind from the loneliness. Having EHS meant that I was unable to do any of those things if I didn't want to exacerbate my symptoms. So, my nights were mostly spent in bed, in silence. Days that I didn't have treatments (Sundays) were spent alone in bed or sitting outside in my backyard staring at the birds. I couldn't do anything at all that involved electronics and the damage from my symptoms made it difficult to do pretty much anything else. I tried reading, but it hurt my eyes. I tried making puzzles but my hands were too shaky and I couldn't concentrate. I even tried writing and that never panned out. The only thing I could do was sit and stare.

I felt as if I were trapped in my body, watching the whole world pass by. It was as if I blinked and the next month flew by. I had completed all of the treatments and yet I was still sick. My doctor prescribed additional at home treatments and sent me packing. I remember thinking, " I thought all of this was going to get me better, why am I not better?" The doctor assured me once again that I was on the right track but honestly, I didn't feel that way. In order to understand just how "beneficial" these treatments were, I started to refer to my health in percentages. Prior to treatment I would have put myself at 0% healthy. After treatment I was around 30% healthy. The treatment did something, but definitely not what I was expecting. I was expecting at least 60% health. However, beggars can't be choosers...

Ketamine

The uncertainty of what to do next really sank in as the next few days passed. I was still sick and starting to lose hope again. What gave me hope again was Ketamine. Arriving at the ketamine office for the first time was extremely comfortable. The owner of the company as well as his staff, were amazing and down to earth. They made me feel right at home by cracking "dad jokes" and talking to me about my interests. I was treated like a person rather than a person who was sick. It was nice.

Ketamine had been recommended by my previous doctor as a way to reduce brain inflammation and brain fog. The treatments lasted approximately 4 hours and always took place in the evening. The office in which the Ketamine was administered was small. It had a waiting room and two treatment rooms. The bathroom was located outside of the office, down the hall. Inside the treatment room was an extra-large brown chair, ottoman, desk/desk chair, a large wooden armoire, a wooden tower with an old school single light bulb lamp, and a red leather guest chair. The guest chair was always filled, unlike before. Due to the fact that ketamine is a hallucinogenic drug, I wasn't allowed to ever drive home and therefore I always had a guest, my new girlfriend.

A month prior to starting ketamine, I had met someone who eventually became my girlfriend. Asking her to drive me to and from my Ketamine appointments made sense at the time. The first day of Ketamine, my girlfriend showed up just as I was feeling the effects of the medicine kick in. Once the Ketamine kicks in most people sleep, I always fought that urge and tried to stay awake in order to try and fully experience what was happening to me. Ketamine was no joke. I hallucinated each time I was treated and apparently always said some really interesting things. None of which I will mention.

In order to receive the full benefits of Ketamine, it was recommended that I complete 5 sessions, back to back. By day 3, I was already feeling my brain start working again. The brain fog was almost gone, and my energy levels were through the roof. Even my EHS symptoms lessened! I completed the final 2 days and had an overall health percentage of 40%.

New Test Results

A few weeks later I received my final test results from the treatment center. The tests showed my previous infection load as well as my current. The results weren't what I was expecting. The numbers had predominantly gone up, meaning my infection load was worse than before. Below are the new test results compared to the previous:

Lyme Disease (the numbers represent the infection load count)

Infection Name	Previous Result	New Result
Anaplasma phagocytophilium	8	32
Babesia divergens	126	24
Babesia microti	26	42
Bartonella bacilliformis	7	48
Bartonella henselae	37	56
Bartonella Quintana	38	115
Borrelia burgdorferi	145	465
Borrelia miyamotoi	47	69
Borrelia recurrentis	9	39
Ehrlichia chaffeensis	123	52
Rickettsia rickettsia	21	60
Chryseobacterium species	133	0
Staphylococcus haemolyticus	159	0
Staphylococcus lugdunensis	6,458	0
Streptococcus anginosus	8,840	0
Streptococus intermedius	13,904	0
Streptococcus urinalis	41,766	0
Veillonella atypica	423	0

Mold

Mold Mycotoxins	Previous Result	New Result
Aflatoxin-M1 (Aspergillus)	3.50 ng/g	3.5 ng/g
Ochratoxin A (Aspergillus)	11.41 ng/g	25.75 ng/g
Mycophenolic Acid (Penicillum)	255.84 ng/g	82.45 ng/g
Verrucarin A (Stachybotrys)	5.25 ng/g	0 ng/g
Chaetoglobosin A (Chaetomium globosum)	67.19 ng/g	76.89 ng/g

As far as the environmental toxin test results go, I only took the original test and chose not to take it again for new results mainly because it was outrageously priced. I also assumed that if the results of the Lyme and Mold tests were as bad as they were the second time around, then my environmental toxin test would likely be the same.

It was a shock for me to see that even after treatment, my infection loads went up. I remember being scared that I was going to be sick for the rest of my life, dealing with illnesses that nobody understands and that my family doesn't believe in.

Meeting Her

Dating was the last thing on my mind, then I met her. Being with her made me forget that I was sick.

We met fatefully towards the end of my first summer in Arizona. She was the very first person in my personal life that I could talk to without being judged, or made to feel crazy. She listened to my symptoms, and even made suggestions. Her suggestions were held high due to the fact that she was not only someone I trusted, but a Naturopathic Doctor. It was as if the Universe or some higher power was telling me that everything was going to be okay by placing her in my life.

The long list of what was wrong with me was suddenly being tackled by two people rather than one. I had a partner that was not only willing to help, but wanted to. She made me a priority and made my illness her own. I was no longer afraid of what was going to happen next because she was there with me.

Not knowing a whole lot about EHS or Lyme Disease, we spent hours each night talking about the techniques I'd tried as well as the treatments I'd done. Her face seemed to be permanently fixed in a state of shock as we spoke. She was shocked that after everything I had done to get better, I still wasn't. She soon knew everything I knew about my chronic illness and discussing possible solutions was more like a brain storming session.

The first thing she worked on was my diet. Remember before how I thought my diet was amazing? Well it wasn't. At that point, my diet changed, and so did my health. I cut all sugar, gluten, dairy, and meat out of my diet. Something that I had thought I was doing up until meeting her. Although I never enjoyed the foods I was eating, the fact that I was seeing improvements in my overall health was all that mattered.

Exosomes

From what I understood, Exosome treatment was necessary if I wanted to heal from Lyme disease. My body's cells were in a poor state and drastic measures were necessary. Apparently, the cells within the body replicate themselves on a constant basis, while eliminating dead cells and birthing new ones. If the cells in which they are replicating from are in a poor state, then the new cells will be as well. That is where Exosome treatment comes in. Exosomes are new, fresh cells that are introduced into the body. Rather than the body replicating the cells that are in a poor state, the body replicated from the Exosomes.

The treatment took 4 hours and was administered in a private room at the Lyme and Cancer treatment center through an IV. Being that they were unprepared for my scheduled appointment, I was forced to wait 2 hours prior to actually starting the treatment. This was in order for the Exosomes to thaw out after being frozen for transport. I felt no different after the 4 hour treatment ended and was told that it would take up to 9 months to see results.

Tackling EHS

Months later, while researching EMFs, I came across an article discussing AC Electric fields and their effects on the human body. Prior to this, I knew about EMFs but only enough to know that they were bad and causing me pain. So, I set out on a mission to become as knowledgeable on EMFs as I could, and I did.

The first step was purchasing a legitimate EMF meter. The discoveries made during that first day playing with the EMF meter were ones that ultimately saved my life. I knew exactly where the problem areas were in my house and did everything I could to eliminate them. No matter what I did, the problem areas couldn't be fixed and therefore I moved.

I moved to a new house in Arizona a week later and began my research on EMFs again. The first thing I did upon moving into my new home was measure the EMFs. While making measurements I learned which areas to avoid. The fact that I had to avoid areas in my house didn't sit well with me so I brainstormed possible solutions. That night I couldn't sleep and remember having hot and cold flashes that prevented me from doing any further research. The next day I started to recognize a pattern. Each night, my symptoms would get worse than they were during the day. This to me, was a pattern. A pattern that solved the question "what was wrong with me?"

One night I decided to shut the power off to my bedroom and turn off my Wi-Fi. I fell asleep instantly and remember waking up feeling like a completely different person. It was confusing and satisfying at the same time. The vibrations in my body had stopped, my brain fog was nearly gone, and a number of my other symptoms seemed nonexistent. "Did I just solve Lyme Disease?" was the main thought in my head at the time. The transformation was so incredible that I spent the next hour in silence, trying to figure out what had happened. Not fully understanding what my 80% health status meant, I set out on a journey for answers.

Body Voltage

Somehow, I came to the conclusion that the answer had to do with body voltage. So, I fashioned a meter for detecting body voltage out of a multimeter and began testing myself around the house. Using my body as a meter was the best decision I could have made. Your body voltage should essentially be zero and when it isn't, your cells enter into an excited state. This prevents healing from occurring on many levels.

Walking around the house with my body voltage meter, I watched the numbers jump from 0 to well over 4,500 millivolts (4.5 volts). The craziest part about all of this is that the vibrations in my body as well as a majority of my symptoms would disappear when my body voltage remained under 100 millivolts. Each time it exceeded 100 millivolts my symptoms would come back; like a light switch I was able to turn my symptoms on and off.

Measuring myself lying in bed with the power turned on to my room, my body voltage was well over 5,000 millivolts (5 volts). No wonder I wasn't sleeping! I was bathing myself in a sea of electricity nightly, a time in which my body was supposed to be healing. Turning off the power to my room made a significant difference in my body voltage (1,500 millivolts). Knowing that number was still high, I did everything I could to make my body voltage in bed less than 100 millivolts.

The final solution was one I never would have thought of if it weren't for my girlfriend. While brainstorming we decided to "ground" the bed. This was done by connecting a grounding cable to my box spring, under the bed, and then plugging the other end into the ground portion of a wall outlet. That simple fix dropped my body voltage to 48 millivolts in bed. That night I slept a solid 8 hours, which was the first time I had slept more than a few hours a night in years.

Figuring out how to keep your body voltage below 100 millivolts is a lot harder than it seems. There are EMFs all around us and our bodies act like antennas, picking up stray voltage wherever we go. Although my health was predominately at 80%, whenever I would leave the house, my symptoms would flair up immediately. There wasn't a single place I could go that didn't have some sort of EMFs effecting my body. So, I stopped going outside of my house in order to have some control over the amount of EMF exposure.

As long as I avoided EMFs, my symptoms seemed to be nonexistent. However, there was no way that I was content with living out my life this way. I decided to order as many books on EMFs that I could (rather than using the internet to conduct research) and began expanding my knowledge even more on EMFs. Reading was all that I could do while keeping my body voltage below 100 millivolts. I had to read in a specific spot in my house that had been tested numerous times at around 77 millivolts. Anywhere else and my symptoms would start acting up.

EMF Challenges

After a month of living that way, my symptoms seemed to come back all of a sudden. I remember being extremely confused, thinking "I thought I solved this, what's happening?" It was confusing, but after reading every book I could get ahold of on EMFs I was able to determine that the problem was no longer within my house, but outside. There was nothing that I could do about the exterior EMFs penetrating my walls and entering my body. My theory was confirmed upon purchasing an additional meter that was capable of measuring outside EMF sources as well as pinpoint their exact location.

I would typically feel fine throughout the day sitting in my low body voltage area, reading. However, around 6:00pm every night like clockwork, my symptoms would come back. Even if I were sitting in that exact spot, with extremely low body voltage. Once again, I noticed a pattern.

What was happening was simple: my neighbors would be gone all day at work, not using their home electronics. Once they arrived home, at 6:00pm, they would begin using their electronics. Their electronics weren't anything out of the ordinary. Just television, Wi-Fi, and the occasional phone call. Little did they know, the EMFs from their devices were penetrating through their house, into mine and eventually into my body. This continued night after night until I couldn't take it anymore and decided to try and find somewhere, anywhere, on this earth that was EMF Free for people like me. No such place existed. There was one place though, a small town, which was a "radio silence zone" that seemed to be a safe haven for other people experiencing similar symptoms.

With moving there not an option and nowhere else in the world that was EMF Free, I decided to build an EMF proof tent. I purchased a single person "changing room" tent as well as EMF protection fabric and tape. The next few days I spent outfitting the interior of the tent with full EMF protection. The results were spectacular. Upon entering the tent, I could feel my symptoms lessen even more than before. It was like a dead zone inside the tent. No cell service, no symptoms, and no problems. Well, one problem remained. I had to get out of the tent eventually.

Exiting the tent was painful. I would spend hours inside it, reading or just thinking and when I would exit, my symptoms would come back instantly. The rush of symptoms flooding back made me pass out on numerous occasions. Sitting in the tent became somewhat scary after that and therefore was only used for emergencies. I remember thinking " I solved my illness, but at what cost?"

At that point I no longer believed that I had Lyme Disease, and knew for a fact that the mold had been out of my body for some time. My theory was that it was only Electromagnetic Hypersensitivity (EHS) left to beat. I knew then that living an EMF free lifestyle was what needed to be done more than ever in order to regain my health. I also stopped taking all oral antibiotics and any of the other medications prescribed to me by the Lyme and Cancer treatment center.

COVID-19

Towards the end of my first year in Arizona, a pandemic hit the world. The pandemic was Covid-19 and it left the world experiencing life through the eyes of the chronically ill. Like having a chronic illness, the world was forced to stop, quarantine and adapt. This time period was difficult for me.

Stores were out of toilet paper, paper towels, water bottles, and even hand sanitizer. However, the lack of groceries was not what was difficult for me. It was the fact that everyone was now at home, using their electronics all day, rather than only after 6:00pm. My healing took a turn for the worse and my body voltage remained well over 100 millivolts. I knew it was EMF related but couldn't control my neighbors Wi-Fi use.

The quarantine had officially knocked my healing percentage back from 80% to 60% and there was nothing I could do. I tried sitting in my EMF tent, but it was no longer strong enough to block out the constant parade of neighboring EMFs. I tried wrapping myself up in faraday cloth, but it left me feeling overheated. Nothing I tried worked, and it left me feeling like giving up.

The first month of quarantine seemed to drag on. Being in pain from symptoms 24/7 made seconds feel like hours and days seem like lifetimes. At any given point of the day, I could tell which neighbors were home, all from their EMF usage. My backyard no longer was safe, and going downstairs even for a moment made me feel as if I were going to faint. I could feel myself losing the battle against EMFs, and there was nothing I could do about it. The constant background readings on my radio frequency meter in my home were:

1. Backyard- 700 µW/m^2
2. Downstairs- 460 µW/m^2
3. Upstairs- 180 µW/m^2

As you can see, there was nowhere in my home that was safe for my body to heal. For those of you who are unaware of safe levels of radio frequencies to be around, the answer is zero. However, the general recommendation found while researching is to remain under 1 µW/m^2 in order to avoid any damage to your body on a cellular level.

Finally, after months of the world being on lockdown the quarantine ended. This was a joyous day for me, because I thought my healing would resume. I was wrong. Many people had lost their jobs due to their company's they once worked for going out of business. Or the company itself had new guidelines which meant less staff members. This resulted in all of my neighbors remaining jobless and my healing process remaining on pause.

Mustering up as much strength as I could, one day I decided to leave my house to see if it were just my neighborhood that was high in EMFs. I brought my radio frequency meter with me, and got into my car. While driving I noticed something that I had not noticed before, more cell towers. From the moment I saw my first cell tower, my meter didn't fall below 50 µW/m2 and spiked to well over 2,000 µW/m2 every 30 seconds. There were literally hundreds more cell towers than before the quarantine had begun. This led me to believe that my neighborhood was not the only one experiencing high levels of EMFs.

After approximately 15 minutes of driving, I turned around and headed back home to document my findings. However, upon getting home, I felt worse than I had in a long time with a health percentage of 10%. My brain fog was back, my body was vibrating from my feet up to my head, I was extremely agitated, my breathing became labored, and walking became difficult. Not being sure if it was due to my exposure outside of my home while driving or inside, I decided to take some Tylenol and take a nap.

After waking up from my nap, my girlfriend arrived home and I discussed my findings with her. Her response was "we need to move". She could see just how bad of shape I was in and offered her assistance as well as telling me that we had to move every 20 minutes. In my head though, I had given up already. I made peace with the fact that I was going to live like this forever and replied "no let's wait to move until I get better." In that response, she could tell I had given up and to her, that wasn't an option.

This is when she decided to make it her personal mission to learn the science behind what was happening to my body. Since she was a naturopathic doctor, the science portion came easier to her than it did for me. She eventually figured out a portion of what was occurring on a cellular level, and began researching supplements to fix the damage that had been done by EMFs.

It wasn't enough to simply remove myself from EMFs, I had to repair the damage on the inside of my body as well. At this point I began researching supplements that other people suffering from EHS had taken.

EMF Free Community

While conducting research on EHS and what supplements others have taken to cure themselves, I came across a statistic that revealed that approximately 3% of the world's population suffered from EHS and it's only going to get worse. Which meant that there are millions upon millions of people going through the same struggles that I have. That statistic haunted me for quite some time, until the idea to build an EMF Free community came to me.

It would be a place for people suffering from EHS could go to in order to heal but most of all somewhere where we would be safe. One of the main things that I haven't felt in the world today is safe and therefore creating an atmosphere of safety was the top priority. Other than safety, it would provide belief. Having individuals believe me that I have been struggling with an invisible illness has been difficult. Not that them believing me was something that I needed, but it would have been nice to know that I wasn't alone. At the EMF free community, people would know that they weren't alone, and would be able to have a community of people that would be there for them.

From that point forward I decided to create a plan for

an EMF Free community that went like this:

1. Step 1- Find a large piece of land away from man-made EMFs.
2. Step 2- Build an EMF proof community center containing a doctor's office, restaurant, gym and treatment rooms.
3. Step 3- Build individual EMF proof homes that people suffering from EHS could move into while healing.
4. Step 4- Train doctors on EHS and EMFs and hire them to work inside the community center.
5. Step 5- Train a team of home inspectors that would EMF proof individuals' homes after leaving the community or providing them with the training they need to do it on their own once home.
6. Step 6- Train a chef on a sugar free, gluten free, dairy free menu.
7. Step 7- Train a personal trainer on how to work out people suffering from EHS.
8. Step 8- Open an EMF Free community by following steps 1-7 in places all over the world.

Following the above steps would lead to the creation of a safe haven for those suffering from EHS. Individuals would not only have a place to let their bodies heal from the damage caused by EMFs, but a place for them to get their lives back. They would also receive treatments from actual doctors who have been trained on EHS and EMFs. Also, everything would be set at an affordable price due to the fact that most people with EHS are unable to work.

I even took this idea as far as to create a daily routine of what a typical day at the EMF Free community would look like. Below is my vision:

1. Prior to arrival an individualized plan will be set for each person. This will be accomplished either through phone or email communication. If that is not possible then an appointment will be set for an in person consultation prior to checking in to the community.
2. Arrive at the community and get checked in by an EMF literate staff member.
3. Receive a welcome packet explaining in detail everything that will occur during their stay. This will include a schedule detailing treatments, meals, activities and appointments. A section on "why" will also be included.
4. You will then be walked to your room by an EHS literate staff member.
5. Once inside your room, the staff member will go over the various details of the room and explain how the room will benefit you. The schedule will also be explained as well as any questions answered.
6. An orientation will be held in the community center once everyone has been checked into their rooms. This will also include a tour of the facility, showing exactly where each treatment or appointment will occur. Staff members will also be introduced.
7. That concludes day one. Each person staying at the community will then retire to their individual rooms.

8. Day two will begin with freshly cooked breakfasts either in the restaurant or in your room.
9. After breakfast, depending on your schedule, you will either meet with your doctor, begin a treatment, enjoy an EMF Free activity, or attend other scheduled appointments.
10. After morning appointments, lunch will be served.
11. After lunch, depending on your schedule, you will either meet with your doctor, begin an additional treatment, enjoy an EMF Free activity, or attend other scheduled appointments.
12. After afternoon appointments, dinner will be served.
13. After dinner, an optional group session will occur. This will be a time for people to sit in a circle and tell their stories or just get to know each other. This is optional because sometimes people prefer solitude.
14. The above daily schedule will occur every day for the first 5 days.
15. Then you will have a two day break from scheduled appointments to do whatever you please within the EMF Free community.
16. After the two day break, schedules will resume again.
17. This will occur for a total time of one month.
18. After you complete your first month at the EMF Free community, you will then meet with your doctor to check in for a one month consultation. At this point you and your doctor will determine if you are at a point where you feel healthy enough to head back

home.
19. Living EMF Free, eating healthy, and receiving treatments for an entire month may be enough for some people to regain their health. If not, then the process would continue for an additional month, followed by a second month check in consultation with your doctor.
20. If you are at a point where you are ready to head home, two options will be presented to you. Option 1- teach you how to recreate the EMF Free environment you have lived in for the past month, or Option 2- have one of our staff members go to your home and do it for you.
21. You leave the community feeling better than you ever have before, equipped with the knowledge necessary to continue living and EMF Free lifestyle.
22. For a set amount of time after leaving, weekly check ins with your doctor are optional.

As you can see, my vision was extremely detailed. I chose to envision exactly what I felt that I needed in order to heal from EMFs. I feel as if it takes a minimum of 4 weeks of EMF Free living and healthy eating to get to a point where you feel better. Sadly, getting out of EMFs in today's world is nearly impossible.

Being EHS myself, it has been extremely difficult trying to get the community started. My struggles began with finding land that was free of man-made EMFs. I would search online, find a parcel of land (typically 40 acres and above), type the address into antennasearch.com and check to make sure there were no cell phone towers anywhere near the land in question. This eliminated 75% of possible land options in Arizona. Then after that, I'd have to eliminate an additional 20% of options because of cost. It was ridiculous how much some of the land options costed and therefore they were eliminated. What was left over was 5% of my initial search and within those options, they were all extremely far from civilization.

Being far from civilization was good because there was definitely no man made EMFs, but bad because it would take hours to get there from any town or airport. The only parcel of land that I could find that fit all of my prerequisites, was located a few miles from a town in Arizona called St. John's.

St. Johns

Heading to St. John's was memorable, to say the least. The morning of the trip began with a high exposure of EMFs which led to an abundance of symptoms. However, I was determined to get there, tour the land, and start a new life away from EMFs. That's not exactly what happened though.

Finding this parcel of land took a lot of effort. It had to be away from technology, away from cell towers, and basically away from everything I once depended on. On top of all the strict requirements for the land, dealing with realtors proved to be a struggle in itself.

Contacting the realtor to tour the land was one of my first setbacks. Remember, EHS restricts the available communication options in order to avoid EMFs. So, I asked the realtor through email to keep our communication strictly through email. He did not comply. I explained to one realtor that I have Lyme Disease and one of my symptoms is a "sensitivity to electronics" and therefore using the phone was not an option. That didn't register with the first realtor, who insisted numerous times for me to call him. Thinking he needed to talk on the phone for some important reason, I agreed to a phone call. This was not something that I wanted to do, but I did it.

The call was painful. I felt my entire body begin to vibrate and my head begin to spin. The realtor had no questions, no important information to share, he just wanted to talk on the phone. To this day I don't understand why a simple accommodation of using email to communicate could not be met. Anyways, an appointment to see the land was set for that week.

A day later I received a text message from the realtor saying he needed to speak with me on the phone AGAIN! I insisted on keeping it through email and yet, he persisted. I eventually set up a time to talk to him again over the phone, thinking once again that this call was of some importance. It was not.

The realtor informed me that he was "actually going out of town for a vacation" and needed to reschedule my appointment with an additional realtor. Ridiculous, right? I thought so myself. Rather than explaining that over email, he chose to inconvenience my health and wellness by using a phone call to relay the message. If that weren't enough, he didn't pass along any information about my preference to use email communication to the new realtor and the process started all over again.

The new realtor was worse than the first. He insisted as well that we speak on the phone, so we set an appointment time for that night at 7:00pm. At 7:00pm I called, with no answer. Seconds later I received a text message from him saying "I'll call you right back". So, I sat there, waiting for him to call with my phone off of airplane mode... 10 minutes went by, nothing....20 minutes went by, nothing....after 30 minutes of waiting for him to call me back I decided to send a text message asking if he were going to call. He called that very second, didn't apologize for keeping me waiting, and blurted out "so, what questions do you have for me?" I couldn't believe it! I had already been in email communication with this second realtor and had already strongly insisted that I did not want to speak on the phone. I just wanted to tour the land at my original appointment time. That wasn't an option with this realtor so we set up a date and time two weeks from my original appointment. I informed the realtor that if any further questions or concerns came up on his behalf that I would prefer email communication due to the fact that my phone was on airplane mode 99% of the day.

Two days before my appointment to tour the land came up, I received a text message from the realtor claiming that he forgot our appointment date and time and needed to confirm it with me... I confirmed it but was really upset with how difficult the process had been. Brushing all that off, I looked forward to touring the land and potentially getting my life back.

The land was located in St. John's, Arizona. However, the nearest hotel was an hour away in Show Low, Arizona. So, my girlfriend and I drove down the day before the tour in order to get a feel for the area and make sure it was safe to stay the night (EMF wise). Upon getting to the hotel, I could already feel my symptoms flaring up, but I kept quiet. I didn't want my girlfriend to know that I was in pain and tried my best to hide it from her. Why I did that, I don't know, maybe pride?

Noticing that I was in pain, my girlfriend forced me to leave the hotel mid-day and head to St. John's to see if I could get some EMF relief. Smart move on her behalf because the second we exited the town of Show Low, my painful symptoms began to fade away.

We entered the small town of St. John's, and was immediately pulled over by a police officer for a "failure to use my turn signal". Which in my opinion was not the reason why we were pulled over. I have California license plates, and this was a small town, you do the math.

The police officer ended up being extremely nice and after explaining my situation he let me off with a warning. Not before my girlfriend invited him to visit the land in the future for a barbecue(if we ended up liking it). The officer even knew the realtor we were going to be meeting with the next day and gave us directions on how to get to the land. It ended up being a good thing that we were pulled over because without his directions, we would have never found the entrance to the land.

Entering the 36,000 acre property felt somewhat scary but exciting at the same time. The long dirt road went on for miles as we drove deeper and deeper into the mountains. There was literally nobody out there, just a bunch of cows, trees, and mountains. The further we got into the property, the more my symptoms disappeared. At one point we stopped the car, got out and I remember feeling like a completely different person. All of my symptoms were gone, I was 100% better and 100% myself. It was a definite eye opening moment for my girlfriend who saw the change before her very eyes. She was happier than I was, not kidding.

We spent the next few hours driving around the vacant land with the windows down, loving life and talking about how weird EMFs and EHS is. Eventually, the sun started to set and since I was "all better" we decided to head back to Show Low to sleep for the night. That was a really bad idea, and I'll tell you why.

Earlier when we were at the hotel, my symptoms were bad, but nobody else was there. That night when we arrived, it was packed, which meant EMFs were high and I felt them immediately. Not only did I feel them, but they took me to a dark place. I felt my entire body shutting down, from my eyes going blurry, to my heart racing at 120 BPM, and to me fighting from losing consciousness. The vibrations I normally felt when exposed to high levels of EMFs was nothing compared to feeling like I was going to die. Rather than wake my girlfriend up, I chose to try and "fight through the pain". That was dumb and I mean really dumb.

I couldn't sleep in the bed because my body voltage was over 800mV when laying on it. The entire room had radio frequency levels 100 times higher than I was normally used to, and that was after unplugging everything. It was extremely high everywhere I went, so I sat in the middle of the room in a chair with my feet lifted off the ground and was wrapped up completely in multiple layers of faraday cloth.

Even after doing all of that, it seemed as if nothing worked. The EMFs were so much higher than I was used to and literally none of my protective clothing/equipment worked to stop them. It was at that point that I realized it was 5G.

Not being able to think or really speak due to the pain, I remember grunting a lot. Which is what I think woke my girlfriend up. After that was a bit of a blur. I do remember her telling me that she felt vibrations in her body while lying on the bed. Something that she had never said before. Even though she was feeling the vibrations that I had felt before, I didn't believe her. I know what you're thinking, "how could I not believe her when I felt the same thing?" I think it had something to do with my symptoms in that moment. I had a difficult time trusting myself, so trusting her was difficult.

The reason why it was so difficult to trust myself/her was because of the psychological impact this process had taken on me. In that moment I thought she was mocking me or saying that she felt what I was feeling in order to "be there for me". I was wrong, and for that I am sorry.

Back to the story. After our brief conversation about her feeling the vibrations, she fell back asleep and I continued to keep my pain/symptoms to myself. Once again, I don't know why I did that, pride I'm assuming.

An hour or so later, my girlfriend woke up again and this time she knew something was seriously wrong with me. I could barely speak, but was able to muster up enough strength to answer her when she asked if we should leave. At that point, we packed up all of our stuff in the hotel and got into my car. Not having anywhere to go, my girlfriend insisted that we drive back to St. John's and sleep in my car, on the land.

As we drove further and further away from Show Low and the hotel, my symptoms once again began to disappear. However, this time was different. Even though the immediate symptoms related to being in extreme EMFs was gone, the affect it left on my body was still there. I felt like I had been in a fight and my whole body was in pain. Being out of EMFs wasn't enough, but I didn't know that at the time. My body was just done fighting and wanted to shut down for the night.

We slept in my car that night, but only for a few hours. At around 4:00am I couldn't take the pain anymore and woke my girlfriend up. We decided to head back home for me to recover from the exposure and hopefully be able to get back to where I was before the trip to St. John's. She texted the realtor from my phone explaining that I wasn't feeling well and that we would have to reschedule the appointment. It was early still, so we didn't receive a response.

Driving back was worse than driving to St. John's. It was as if my body or nerves had been rubbed raw and every single cell tower we passed caused me excruciating pain. It wasn't just the cell towers though; it was everything EMF related that caused me pain. Passing by a car where the driver was clearly on their phone, made my head pound and my heart race.

The weirdest thing happened while driving back. Once we were back near home, the pain seemed to dissipate and I remember saying "whoa I feel different, I knew it was 5G." Even though I didn't know exactly why my pain had lessened, it made me feel better to think it was because I was out of 5G.

After that, it took approximately 2 days for me to get back to "normal". For those two days I stayed inside my room, avoided any EMFs that I could, stayed wrapped up in faraday cloth, ate healthy, drank plenty of water, and took my supplements. Surprisingly, all of that worked wonders. I still felt like something was off though and chalked it up to the after effects of being exposed to high levels of EMFs.

At some point while away, my neighbors either started working again, or got new jobs because the EMF levels at my home became tolerable once again. The constant background radio frequency levels were now:

1. Upstairs: .5-3 µW/m2
2. Downstairs: 1-5 µW/m2

These levels stayed within that range and periodically would pulse to higher levels, mainly coming from the smart meters surrounding my home. Using my radio frequency blocking blankets, I was able to lower my exposure to near zero within my home. Although the levels were now something I could tolerate, my mind at this point was suffering. I felt trapped. Trapped in the sense that I was never going to get better and even if I did, I wouldn't be able to leave my home. My mind went to some dark places for a while and thoughts of suicide were among the darkest. However, I kept all of my darkness inside of me and pretended that I was okay, even though I was not.

New Supplements

After St. John's, my spirits were low but I knew deep within me that something was missing. Something that was overlooked. So, I began researching and re reading books I had already read, hoping the answers I was seeking would be revealed. In my research I found an individual who claimed to have cured himself of EHS, and a supplement he used to do so was "Olive leaf extract".

Without looking up what it was exactly, I decided to order a variation of the supplement called "Olivirex". After receiving it in the mail and reading how many to take, I took my first dose. Within approximately 1 hour, my brain fog had lifted more than it had in the past but honestly, I thought it was just a coincidence. I knew that I needed to consistently take the supplement for a few days before real results would surface. To my surprise, after 5 days of taking the new supplement, my brain fog and vibrations in my body had significantly reduced.

Not knowing if it was all in my head or if I was truly seeing results, I decided to experiment on myself. Risky, I know, but I figured "it's either this or keep assuming it was working." My experiment was simple, take the supplements one day, track my symptoms, and then don't take the supplements another day and track those symptoms.

While taking the supplements, I had noticeable decreases in brain swelling, brain fog, vibrations in my body, and an increase in overall well-being. My health percentage was a consistent 80%, with random spikes of up to 90%. Some moments I would feel so amazing that I would forget that I were sick...seriously.

The one and only day I chose not to take the supplement (for experimental purposes only), started out normal. My health percentage was still 80% and my symptoms were at a minimal. The mistake I made that day was changing my environment. The day before, while taking the supplement, I stayed home. The day I did not take the supplement, I felt so good that I decided to leave my house.

That horrible idea ruined my experiment because I was unable to tell if it were my exposures (EMFs) or lack of the supplement that caused my symptoms to come back.

While out at the store, my brain fog as well as my other symptoms came back instantly. So, I returned home and my health status had dropped to 50%. After that, I became frustrated with the thought that I truly couldn't leave my house if I wanted to get better.

With my experiment ruined and my symptoms back, I decided to do something that was unlike my character. I asked for help.

My girlfriend, being a Naturopathic Physician and extremely knowledgeable on supplementation, was naturally the only person that came to mind. She figured out an exact supplement regimen that would eventually lead to my recovery.

The supplement regimen was as follows:

1. Olivirex (2 pills, twice a day)
2. SafeCell (2 pills, twice a day)
3. Designs for Health Twice Daily Essential Packets (4 pills, twice a day)
4. NAC 900mg (1 pill, once a day)
5. L-Arginine (2 pills, once a day)
6. Mitochondria ATP (2 pills, once a day)

These supplements however, were not "store bought" meaning that they were only able to be purchased through specialty labs. The reason for this as explained by her, was because store bought supplements are unreliable. They apparently use "fillers" and "cheaper alternatives" to the actual supplement listed on the front of the bottle. In order to ensure that I was receiving the actual supplement my body needed, she opted for reputable companies that guaranteed what was in the bottle. Not all companies do that.

After a full week of taking the new supplement regimen as well as not leaving my house, I felt like a completely different person. I felt so good in fact, that I thought I was cured and began planning a trip to Sedona in order to attempt to look at land for an EMF Free community.

Sedona

Attempt number two at finding an EMF Free location was in Sedona, Arizona. It was a lot more expensive than St. John's but my thoughts were "you can't put a price on being healthy" and I'm sure a lot of people would agree.

Driving to Sedona was beautiful but its beauty was quickly overshadowed by the new cell towers located inside the town. One of the new cell towers was less than 100 feet off the main strip where the shops were. The fact that there were cell towers in the town surprised me, because I knew Sedona was one of the first cities to ban Smart Meters. So naturally, I thought if they were smart enough to ban smart meters, there's no way they would ever allow cell towers. Once again, I was wrong.

Being the tough guy that I am, I decided to try and ignore the pain I felt from the new cell tower and go to a restaurant for lunch with my girlfriend. Being that there were new rules and regulations in place due to Covid-19, the restaurant didn't have menus. Instead there were these barcode looking things on our table and the waitress informed us that we needed to scan it with our cell phone to get the menu. That was frustrating because my girlfriend and I didn't bring our phones.

After explaining how we didn't have our phones, paper menus were provided and we were able to order our lunch. The conversation my girlfriend and I had while waiting for our lunch was about how every single person around us was on their phone. People seriously don't talk to each other anymore, it's weird. Or if they were talking to each other, their eyes would be glued to their cell phones still.

The pain from being around all the cell phones and a few hundred feet from the new cell tower eventually became unbearable, so we finished lunch and decided to head to the hotel to check in.

The check in area at the hotel looked like a bank. Plexiglass extended up from the check in desk to protect the staff from possible infection and lines covered the floor every 6 feet to ensure guests social distanced.

Once checked in, we headed to our hotel room and began doing a full EMF inspection. The main problems found were the dirty electricity, body voltage in bed, and the new Wi-Fi router they had installed by the phone. We were able to lower the dirty electricity levels by installing filters on 7 of the outlets and even disconnected the Wi-Fi router to eliminate the radio frequencies inside the room. The body voltage on the bed however, was very difficult to lower. The bed frame itself was metal, so we grounded that, lowering my body voltage from 350 millivolts to 295 millivolts. The reason we were unable to get our body voltage lower than that was because the mattress itself had metal springs in it. Since we couldn't cut open the mattress and ground the metal springs, 295 millivolts was the lowest we were able to get it.

Then after completing our EMF inspection, more guests began checking into the rooms surrounding us. At that point they all connected to Wi-Fi, used their phones, and started watching television. Instantly the radio frequency meter shot up to levels well above safe limits and my body felt like it was being suffocated. I felt like my entire body was vibrating from my toes all the way up to my head and no matter where I went inside the room, I couldn't feel any relief.

My girlfriend then took a turn for the worst and was complaining about stomach pain and head pressure. Her thought was that she took too many B vitamins and it was making her feel nauseas. So, I sucked up my pain and tried to be there for her. The only thing we could think of in that moment was to go for a walk and try to see if that helped her. We walked for 20 minutes, away from the hotel, away from cars, and away from people. That seemed to help me because my symptoms almost completely disappeared. I remember telling her that I felt 80% healthy but she was still not feeling well so we found a few rocks and decided to sit and wait.

Sitting there we went through all the supplements she had taken that day and tried to rule out her B vitamin theory. She eventually threw up and because she still wasn't feeling well, we headed back towards the hotel. While walking however, she miraculously felt better so once again we stopped and decided to wait a little longer for her to fully recover.

After recovering some more, we headed into the hotel parking lot. Instantly, I felt a wave of symptoms hit my body and dropped from my previous 80% health status, to 10%. My head was pounding, my heart was beating erratically, I could barely breathe and yet none of that mattered because my girlfriend was experiencing very similar symptoms. Since I wasn't all that comfortable talking about My EHS, I kept trying to think of any other reason why she could be feeling what I was feeling. I remember thinking "could it be food poisoning? Maybe her B vitamin theory is correct. But then I'd have to have taken B vitamins as well and I didn't. She can't be EHS, could she?"

We spent the next hour seriously trying to figure out if somehow she could have become sensitive to EMFs but eventually, we gave up and decided to go pick up some dinner. While driving to pick up food, our symptoms disappeared at the same time. Weird, I know. The thought that she was faking it, did cross my mind but the fact that she spoke out loud telling me her symptoms and then telling me when they disappeared, lined up exactly with what was happening to me.

We returned to the hotel room, ate our dinner, and then my girlfriend fell asleep. I, however, couldn't sleep. My body voltage was way higher than I was used to, and the radio frequencies were pulsing off the charts (confirmed with my meter). I spent the next few hours wrapped in my faraday blankets until eventually I passed out from the pain.

Around 4:30am I woke up feeling like I had been hit by a truck. My entire body was "jittery" and my muscles felt extremely weak. So, I did what I thought would help, and got into the shower to try and soothe the pain away. A little while later my girlfriend noticed I wasn't in bed, went into the bathroom and said "I feel jittery". I couldn't believe it, she literally took the words out of my mouth and doubting her symptoms after that was impossible.

We immediately decided to go out for another walk and try to get away from the high EMF environment. Surprisingly, it worked. The further we got from the hotel, the better both of us felt. After about 30 minutes we headed back into the hotel with a game plan we came up with out on our walk. Our game plan was simple, go get breakfast.

After getting breakfast, her symptoms had disappeared and she was feeling like herself again, and I was at 60% health. We headed back to the hotel once again and once in our room, my girlfriend fell asleep again.

Once awake, we discussed our symptoms and decided that we would go and take a look at the land. After all, that's why we were there in the first place. To look for land to build an EMF Free community. That didn't go so well.

The land had radio frequency readings that were too high for the community to be there, so we packed up our meters and headed back to the hotel. At this point my health percentage was around 10% and I knew I wouldn't be able to make it another night so we packed everything up and left Sedona.

It took approximately 2 days for me to get back to 80% health.

Conclusion

After getting back from my second failed attempt at finding land, I gained a new perspective on life. My perspective was simple, don't give up. Rather than continue to search for land though, I decided to write this book. While compiling my notes and writing the various sections, I came to the conclusion that 80% healthy was the best that I would ever get. It was a sad moment for me because for years I did everything possible that I could think of to get myself back to 100% and yet, I had to settle on the fact that I would never get there.

For days I stopped verbalizing my symptoms to my girlfriend, something that she had grown reliant on because of how good I was at hiding my pain behind a smile. During that time, she had no clue that I felt defeated and had settled on 80% health, or so I thought. Little did I know, she knew I had felt defeated and continued researching the science behind EMFs on her own. She never gave up on the thought that reaching 100% health wasn't possible and eventually made a break through discovery during her research.

One day she came home with a folded piece of paper in her hand, shouting "PARP babe, I figured it out!" The folded piece of paper she was carrying was supposed to be a chart that I would understand, but science was never something I was good at. So, she decided to explain what EMFs were doing to my body on a cellular level, in ways that I understood. Her explanation was as follows:

1. Imagine that you have little workers inside of your body and their main job is to make repairs.
2. Each worker has a set of tools as well as a bucket to carry their tools.
3. Rather than multiple workers inside my body, I only have 1 worker left.
4. On top of only having 1 worker, that worker doesn't have any of the necessary tools to make repairs.
5. When EMFs attack the body on a cellular level, this one little worker heads over to the damage and doesn't have the tools to fix the damage.
6. By sending in the tools through supplements, the worker gains the tools needed to make repairs.
7. Eventually more workers join the crew and begin making repairs with the tools provided by the supplementation.
8. By avoiding EMFs long enough, and supplying the necessary supplements to make repairs, the body is then able to heal on a cellular level.

After her lengthy explanation of what was happening to my body, she followed with "and I know how to fix it." Words that I had never heard come out of her mouth before in regards to EHS. She knew the exact supplementation regimen that my body needed to be on in order to heal the damage that had been done by EMFs. The supplements ordered were as follows:

1. Molecular Hydrogen
2. Tru Niagen Pro 500
3. Magnesium Powder
4. CoQ-10
5. Liposomal Glutathione
6. Nrf2

Within 30 minutes of taking these new supplements, I remember thinking "I need to rewrite my ending, I feel amazing." In that moment I felt 95% healthy and knew she was right about what my body needed. That next morning however, I was woken up to the pain of an excruciating headache. My left eye felt as if it had a knife in it, and my brain felt like it was swollen and going to explode.

Monsoon season in Arizona had started, which meant that I couldn't tell if the headaches were from the change in weather or were an adverse side effect to the new supplements. The headache continued for a few hours, and didn't subside even after taking Tylenol, or icing my head. After the weather cleared up, my headache disappeared. A coincidence that led me to conclude it was the weather and not the new supplements.

For about a week, I continued taking the new

supplements while avoiding EMFs, and my health percentage remained above 90%, even with the weather acting up. If my girlfriend would have given up, I would have never reached 90% health as well as creating my new perspective in life of not giving up. With my health at a minimum of 90%, one night I proposed to my girlfriend and she said yes. If it weren't for her, I would have had no one in my life, and would have given up a long time ago. In a way, she brought me back to life and it is my hope to spend the rest of my life showing her just how grateful I am for her love, patience, support, belief in me, and most of all for her not giving up on me.

All that I truly needed throughout being sick with mold illness, Lyme disease, and EHS was for someone to believe me. Although the illnesses were claimed to be "all in my head" by the people closest to me, I can assure you that they were not, and I went through years of torture to prove it. While the story you have read may seem like a lot, it was merely just a glimpse of what I went through. In the following chapters I attempt to connect the dots regarding what I believe happened to my health, as well as provide an honest look at where I'm at today, the other weird symptoms experienced, and even the various other things I tried in order to regain my health.

Chapter 2

Connecting the Dots

Have you ever heard of the term "connecting the dots"? It's a simple concept that involves going through something and not understanding why you were going through it until later on down the road when you are able to connect the dots. Here is my attempt at connecting the dots.

I believe I was exposed to mold for a prolonged period of time, which weakened my immune system.

Then I contracted Lyme disease and because my immune system was so weak, it took over my body.

After that, my body became so toxic from the mold and Lyme disease that I was unable to detox. Not being able to detox led to the development of Electromagnetic hypersensitivity (EHS).

What cured me was detoxing my body, and then adding beneficial supplements to repair the damage that had been done over the years of continuing to expose myself to EMFs. By aiding my bodies detoxification process and adding the beneficial supplements, I was able to cure myself of mold illness, Lyme Disease, and almost of EHS.

I wasn't able to connect the dots until going through everything and truly understanding what was happening to my body. I needed to start trusting my instincts because let's face it, I had been right about everything I was experiencing the entire time. Like most people suffering from an invisible illness, I stopped trusting myself because my illness wasn't something that was accepted.

Looking back now, I am glad that I went through everything that I did. Why? It made me stronger mentally, and it made me open my eyes to a completely different world.

The difficulties I went through are ones that can be avoided, and my goal is to help others avoid them. Below I've listed out the treatments, supplements, and lifestyle changes that I feel were the most helpful at conquering this invisible illness. I am not recommending that you do as I've done, I can't do that, or I'll get in trouble. I'm simply just showing you what I would do if I were just now exhibiting signs and symptoms related to mold, Lyme, or EHS...do whatever you want with the information.

Step 1- Get out of EMFs. If that's not possible, make your living environment as low tech as possible.

I don't use Wi-Fi, I don't have anything plugged in

inside my home except for my refrigerator, and the power to my bedroom is always off (turned off at breaker box). My bed has been grounded and my body voltage remains below 100mV at all times inside my home. Keeping body voltage as close to zero as possible is crucial to the healing process.

I also avoid going out unless absolutely necessary. This is due to the fact that I can't control the outside environment and wherever I go there seems to be a constant bombardment of EMFs. Which I've learned sets you back in the healing process. The longer I go without exposing myself to EMFs, the faster I heal.

As far as my cell phone goes, I try to avoid using it as much as possible and keep it on airplane mode 99% of the day. Using the screen time application, I am able to monitor just how much time I actually use my phone. The only thing I don't like about that application is that it doesn't differentiate between being on airplane mode or not. For those of you thinking "how do people get ahold of you if your phones on airplane mode all the time?", my answer is simple: they don't. I typically turn my phone off of airplane mode once a day to check my email and text messages, then respond accordingly. It may be difficult to get ahold of me in emergency situations, but I'm working on that. My plan for the future is to get a corded landline for emergency purposes. However, I have no friends, so who is going to be calling me? I'm in no rush as of now.

Other than that, anything that sends a signal or plugs into a wall, I don't use. This is strictly for healing purposes and not because I dislike technology. While the body is healing, technology (EMFs) has proven to slow the process of repairing my body on a cellular level. Without any EMFs in my life, my body is able to heal itself naturally and as intended. If I would have trusted myself originally, I wouldn't have gone to the Lyme and Cancer treatment center and wasted months on useless treatments. Avoiding EMFs is free and much more affective.

The top 5 things that I would do in order to lower my EMF exposure are as follows:

1. Turn off or unplug Wi-Fi
2. Cut unnecessary power at breaker box to house
3. Turn off cell phones (airplane mode may not work as intended)
4. Get rid of all Bluetooth enabled devices. Even when they are off, they put off extremely high levels of RF radiation
5. Get rid of all "smart devices"

Step 2- Change your diet and up your water intake. You'd be surprised at how difficult this step actually is.

I don't eat anything with added sugar. Sugar feeds the bad stuff inside your body and contributes to its growth. Therefore, by eliminating sugar, you eliminate growth.

I drink only Mountain Valley water in the glass bottle because of two reasons: 1- it's in glass rather than plastic which can mess with the quality of the water. Think of your plastic water bottle sitting outside on a hot day. Do you think like me and wonder if the heating effect on the plastic causes it to bleed into the water? I feel more comfortable knowing my water is plastic free. 2- the quality of the water you drink is extremely important, and this water is extremely high quality in my opinion. When it comes to quantity of water, I try to drink at least my weight in fluid ounces daily. I weigh about 200lbs, so I try to drink 200 fluid ounces. I know that may seem like a lot, but EMFs dehydrate you on a cellular level and therefore hydration is essential.

My diet isn't all that difficult. I don't eat any processed foods, and try to only eat organic. I tried going vegan for a while, which didn't work out. However, I significantly cut back on the amount of meat I eat, limiting myself to a slice of turkey here and there as well as some bacon in the mornings. The main thing I would say that I changed diet wise is the amount of vegetables I eat. I try to eat as many vegetables daily as I can. Also, I don't eat gluten or dairy. Cutting gluten out of my diet was actually difficult because I love bread, but I noticed a significant difference in my bodies inflammation from not eating gluten. After all this time, I have grown to actually enjoy gluten free bread, and my body has thanked me.

I also don't use the microwave to heat or make any of my meals. This is for two reasons: 1- microwaves put out high levels of radio frequencies that can be measured up to 30 feet away (I've tested this myself by standing in my backyard 30 feet away from my microwave and measuring levels way above safe limits), and 2- microwaving your food, from my understanding, strips the food of a lot of its beneficial nutrients.

Step 3- Basic supplementation. This step played a crucial role in my healing process. Taking basic supplements helps aid your body in the recovery process by providing much needed vitamins and minerals that aren't included in today's food.

The quality of the supplements also plays a crucial role. In the past, I used to purchase supplements from the same stores I bought my groceries at. That was a big mistake as I soon realized when I switched over to better supplements. Where you purchase basic supplements does matter. From my experience, if it's sold in a store where you buy groceries, it's probably not one that contains the best ingredients.

The basic supplements I took were:

1. Designs for Health Twice Daily Essential Packets (multivitamin, fish oil, magnesium, calcium)
2. Klaire Labs Ther-Biotic Complete (probiotic)

Although the basic supplements that I took contained only 5 supplements, they were exactly what my body needed at the time. I still continue to take this basic supplement twice a day, every day.

Step 4- Detox your body. This can be accomplished by doing a detox program involving shakes, detox supplements, as well as completing a colon hydrotherapy regimen. External options include detox baths and dry brushing.

I started my detox process by taking a candida elimination supplement along with weekly colon hydrotherapies. The candida supplements bind/kill the bad stuff inside your gut and the colon hydrotherapies help suck it out of you. The reason why this worked so well for me was because I had high amounts of candida in my stool test. The total time I spent detoxing from candida was about 30 days.

After detoxing from candida, I started a parasite detox program. For this, all I did was switch to parasite supplements rather than candida supplements, while still continuing the weekly colon hydrotherapies.

A weird trick that I learned while taking parasite detox supplements, is that some parasites glow under UV light. So, each time I used the bathroom, I would bring my UV black light in and inspect my stool for parasites. In the beginning, it looked like a bowl of glowing spaghetti, and by the end of the detox the glowing had disappeared. Some colon hydrotherapy units actually have UV lights attached to them.

The total time spent doing the parasite cleanse was 30 days.

After completing the candida and parasite detoxes, I started doing detox protein shakes. These shakes were absolutely disgusting, but they worked. At first, I tried drinking the shakes with just almond milk and the detox powder, which tasted like I was drinking cardboard. Then I started making actual smoothies to try and mask the horrific cardboard flavor. My shakes consisted of a banana, a handful of fresh strawberries, almond milk, and sometimes a few slices of fresh mango. That combination tasted much better, but still had a hint of cardboard flavor.

The detox protein shakes were supposed to detox my liver and my colon, as well as provide my body with vital nutrients and minerals. This definitely occurred. I chose to drink the shakes an hour or so before bedtime because they made me extremely bloated and very tired. Also, it made my bowel movements more intense the morning after taking a shake.

The total time spent doing the detox protein shakes was one shake a day for 12 days. I was supposed to take 2 shakes a day for the final 6 days, but 1 shake was way more than enough for me to see results.

Along with all of the detox treatments above, I also enjoy dry brushing every single day as a way to detox even more. Something that I had to figure out on my own was that while dry brushing, it is best to brush towards the heart. So, no matter where you are brushing on your body, as long as you are brushing in the direction of your heart, you are doing it correctly.

Step 5- Advanced supplementation. This step involves knowing what your body is lacking on a more specific scale. Most individuals need blood tests in order to see exactly what their body needs. However, for me blood tests weren't enough to diagnose what was happening to my body. It took learning what EMFs were doing on a cellular level as well as experimenting through trial and error in order to figure out what worked for me.

The first set of advanced supplements I added on top of my basic supplements were:

1. Olive Leaf Extract (Olivirex)
2. Liposomal Glutathione

After completing a month of taking the above two advanced supplements and tracking how I felt as well as documenting any changes in my symptoms, I added in a second round of new supplements. On top of the basic supplements, Olive Leaf Extract and Liposomal Glutathione, I added the following supplements:

1. Tru Niagen Pro 500
2. Magnesium Powder
3. CoQ-10
4. Nrf2

These supplements made the largest difference for me in overall health and I continue to take them to this day. For me it was obvious to add these supplements due to the fact that EMFs cause DNA damage. By adding in these supplements, my body was able to repair itself on a cellular level.

In order to get the full benefit of the supplements taken, I continue to limit my EMF exposure as well as maintain the lowest body voltage possible. For more information on what each supplement does, please see the supplementation chapter.

Step 6- Additional Treatments. Following the above steps were enough to get me to 95% health. If I would have followed those rather than waste my time listening to people claim they knew what was wrong with me, I believe that I wouldn't have had to go through years of unnecessary treatments and would have healed myself in a matter of months.

In order to maintain this level of health, I continue to do additional treatments and will continue to do them for the rest of my life. That is my choice, because I choose to never go through Mold, Lyme, or EHS ever again.

For brain fog and brain inflammation I went to a Ketamine specialist and received 4 hour Ketamine treatments for a week straight initially. Later on down the road, if I ever felt the brain fog coming back or my brain starting to inflame again, I would schedule a touch up session. After reaching a certain point, my brain no longer needed Ketamine treatment, but if I ever needed to go back, I know that I would be taken care of by the people at the Ketamine treatment center. To be honest, they were the only individuals who I trusted with the treatment itself and would not go to any other treatment center. Ketamine is no joke, and with the wrong people administering the treatment, the entire session could do more damage than good. Also, on a side note, **do not chew gum** while you are receiving the treatment. I learned from experience that it usually ends up all over the place. I had gum in my beard, all over my face, and on my hands. Luckily, the guys at the treatment center were cool about it and cleaned me up while I was still receiving treatment.

Colon hydrotherapies were something that I used for detox purposes throughout the healing process. There was a lot of information that I found online stating that there is no proof that they are good or bad for you. In the beginning that scared me, but after the hundreds that I have received, I can assure you that they had a benefit at detoxing my body. Whenever I feel as if I am a little more toxic than normal and need to detox, I schedule a session and walk out feeling better than I had when I first went in. They only take about 45 minutes and clean out anything in your gut that you weren't able to get out while "using the restroom". This is something that I will continue to do once a month at the very least for the rest of my life.

Cupping was a treatment that I didn't talk about within the "things I've tried" section because there wasn't a whole lot to write about. I purchased a set of personal cups online that are glass and are easy to use. If I am unable to go to a colon hydrotherapy session, the next best spot detox therapy I use is cupping. Cupping is essentially the process of placing glass cups on specific parts of the body that are suctioned in place through heat, they are then left there for a certain duration of time and pull toxins out of your body at the point of suction. The areas where the cups are placed end up looking like circular bruises and typically last for a few weeks. There are also self-cupping cups available online, but I haven't tried those. I prefer glass on my back. In my opinion, cupping is well worth trying in addition to colon hydrotherapies. Both work wonders at detoxing the body.

On rare occasions I will also get acupuncture for stress relief. It doesn't really do anything else besides remove stress for me, so I do it mainly when I am stressed enough to let someone poke me with needles.

Recapping the 6 steps listed above, I have included a basic list below:

1. Get out of EMFs
2. Change your diet and up your water intake.
3. Basic supplementation
4. Detox your body
5. Advanced supplementation
6. Additional treatments

Chapter 3

Where I'm at Now

If you took the time to read my story and didn't just skip to this chapter, then you'll know just how long and hard this journey has truly been. I was able to beat Mold Illness, Lyme Disease, and have almost completely beaten EHS. Yet, there were times I never thought I was going to make it, and even times where I just wanted to give up. Fortunately, that's not who I am. I am an EHS warrior, fighting a battle against an invisible enemy.

For those of you wondering what my daily schedule looks like now, I've included it below. Although it may vary from day to day, this is what my average routine looks like now.

7:00AM- Wake up. My body naturally wakes up at this time without any alarm. I usually wake up feeling well rested and am able to literally "jump out of bed."

7:15AM- Shower and use the restroom. Like

clockwork, my bowel movements come at the same time every day. I also like to take long showers because it's the one place in my house that I feel the best. Possibly because I have clean water thanks to my shower head filter, or because my body voltage is extremely low in the shower.

7:45AM- Breakfast and supplements. I make the same breakfast every day but rely heavily on my fiancé to do the cooking portion. Let me explain that. I make an egg sandwich every day for breakfast (gluten/sugar/dairy free). However, since I avoid EMFs as much as possible, I make everything but the egg. My fiancé cooks the egg after my sandwich has been made and then places the egg on my complete sandwich. That way, I avoid EMFs. Currently, we have an electric stove so I do everything but the actual using of the stove. The sandwich itself isn't the best tasting, but I would much rather eat that and feel better, than eat something that causes me to feel sick afterwards. After eating, I take my mountain of supplements and try to drink at least 20 fluid ounces of water.

8:00AM- Fiancé leaves for work. Due to the pandemic of COVID-19, my fiancés schedule changed and therefore she leaves at 8:00AM rather than earlier in the day. This give me time to have breakfast with her before she leaves for work. After she leaves, I am alone all day. For most of the people that I tell this part to, they act shocked that I am capable of being alone all day without the use of technology. My response is that it really isn't as difficult as you would think.

8:45AM- Reading time. For the next several hours I sit

in a camping chair that has no metal on it and read. If a neighbor of mine goes into their backyard and is on their phone (this happens a lot), I am then forced to get out of my chair in my living room and head to my bedroom in order to avoid the EMFs from their phones. Sometimes all of my neighbors are home an on their phones or using their Wi-Fi, and I am unable to even sit in my living room. If I don't move, I can literally feel the EMFs and my symptoms flair up. If the EMFs are extremely high, I stay in my bedroom wrapped in faraday blankets and try my best to just read. By EMFs, I simply mean the amount of Radio Frequencies and Dirty Electricity.

12:00PM- Lunch time and more supplements. Depending on how I am feeling, I also turn my phone off of airplane mode for a few minutes to check my email and see if anyone has texted me. Usually it's just my fiancé checking in to see how I am doing. Other than that, nobody else texts me or emails me to see how I am doing so I turn my phone back on airplane mode and make lunch. I eat the same thing pretty much every day, but lunch time is a little more difficult for me. Since my fiancé is at work, I have to be the one to use the stove. So, I usually make a gluten free, dairy free, cauliflower pizza. That way I can limit my EMF use by putting the pizza in the oven, setting a timer, and walking away from the kitchen. There are other meals that I eat for lunch, like beans and rice with vegetables in it, but I prefer making a pizza. It makes me feel like I am eating a normal meal, even if it tastes nothing like a real pizza. After eating, I take more supplements and drink an additional 20 fluid ounces. By this point I've already drank around 60 fluid ounces of water for the day.

1:00PM- Back to reading. I continue to read and avoid EMFs by either being in my bedroom or living room, depending on if my neighbors are still home. If they are gone, I sometimes sit outside and read. However, this has become increasingly difficult with the new cell towers that have been put up in my area. It makes sitting outside painful depending on the time of day. Also, with COVID-19 more of my neighbors are home during the week and therefore sitting outside becomes difficult.

2:00PM- Dry brushing. I try to dry brush at least once a day. At least on the areas that are exposed and not covered by EMF protection clothing. If doing only the exposed areas isn't enough for me to feel some relief, I take an additional shower at this time and dry brush my entire body. Depending on the day, I may even take a detox bath at this time and read in the bathtub with my mold candles going in the background.

3:00PM- Mail check. Being that I'm trapped inside all day, with no connection to the outside world, I try to go outside at least once. If it's too painful to sit in my backyard, I wait until around 3:00PM to walk outside to my mailbox and check the mail. While walking to my mailbox, I pass by at least 10 smart meters (one of which is my own), and therefore I really have to be feeling good symptom wise if I want to make that walk. There's no way to walk where I can avoid the smart meters either, trust me I've tried.

3:10PM- Snack time. I usually get hungry around this time and make myself a protein shake. If, however, my symptoms are flared from my walk or for some other reason, I chose not to use my "magic bullet" blender in order to avoid making my symptoms worse with additional exposures. If that's the case, I eat these seaweed snacks that are actually pretty good or make myself a gluten free, dairy free, sandwich. At this point I've drank about 100 fluid ounces of water.

3:30PM- Reading and writing. Sometimes rather than read, I'll write random stories down on a pad of paper just to keep my mind guessing. Reading all day, every day, can get a little boring so writing is a good way to mix things up. Remember, I don't use any technology throughout the day. So that means: no cell phone, no television, no internet, and nothing else that can emit EMFs.

4:30PM- Cleaning. Since I am a little OCD when it comes to my house, I clean a lot. Cleaning also helps pass the time. I do the dishes, mop the floor, wipe my countertops, and even reorganize furniture (if I have the energy). Also, depending on how I'm feeling I'll also do the laundry. The laundry is a little tricky though because it requires the use of EMFs, so if I'm going to do laundry I have to be as far away from the washer and dryer as possible while they are running. Otherwise, I'll cause a symptom flare up. If my house isn't clean, it bothers me, so I spend about an hour a day doing this. Besides, my fiancé loves coming home to a clean house and I like that I can do at least one thing every day to make her happy.

5:30PM- Back to reading. I read wrapped up in faraday blankets until my fiancé gets home from work, which is usually when all my neighbors get home as well.

6:00PM- Dinner time. Once my fiancé is home, we make dinner together. I usually do what I can, while avoiding EMFs, and she does the rest. If the stove or oven is involved, she takes over completely. I'm very fortunate to have someone who understands EHS and is willing to help the way she does. Dinner is always something extremely healthy. She makes a bunch of meals that surprisingly taste good, even for being healthy. One of my favorites that she makes involves cauliflower and it's really good. Another favorite of mine is black beans, rice, and a bunch of vegetables all mixed together. All of which are freshly prepared and never from frozen bags. The microwave is never used. While eating dinner, we sit and talk to each other. No technology is used. Most people I know, struggle with this part of the day because they are so used to watching television while they eat. We don't. We sit and talk about anything and everything. It's really nice.

7:00PM- Fun time. If I'm feeling good enough, and my neighbor's technology use isn't affecting me, we usually watch a DVD. Using an older DVD player that I inspected myself with my various meters, and connected to a television that isn't "smart" (meaning that it doesn't connect to Wi-Fi), the readings are all below safe limits. I still wrap myself up in my faraday blanket and wear my blue light blocking glasses as an extra precaution. I also light my mold candles throughout the house and do not use any other source of light. If we don't watch a DVD, we play a game called "dominos" or even just sit and talk.

8:30PM- Bed time and supplements. It may seem early but this is the time of day I go to bed. On occasion, my fiancé and I will stay up in bed and talk for a little while. No more than an hour. So technically, sometimes we go to bed around 9:30PM, but never later. Also, I take my detox supplements for the night and finish up my 150-200 fluid ounces of water for the day. In bed, I sleep with faraday sheets, a faraday pillow case, two faraday blankets, a faraday beanie, full faraday protection clothing, my faraday taped noise cancelling headphones, my power shut off to my bedroom (it's actually shut off 24/7), and my bed grounded. I fall asleep within 2 minutes of closing my eyes and for the past month I've been sleeping completely through the night. Also, I dream now. Something I hadn't done in years.

Now you know what a typical day's routine looks like for me. It's definitely an extremely boring lifestyle but that's not a big deal for me. I'd rather be living this boring lifestyle than not living at all. Today I'm actually able to communicate without brain fog, read without forgetting each sentence, and function as normally as possible within my house. On average I feel around 90% healthy, which is amazing considering where I was at before.

My goal for the future is to move but to be completely honest with you, I'm scared. I'm scared because there aren't a lot of options for people suffering with EHS. I mean, I could move to West Virginia and live in the radio silence zone but come on, that's not fair. It's not fair that there's nowhere to go in this world (besides West Virginia) that's completely free of EMFs.

All of the houses I've looked at are equipped with smart meters, which also makes things difficult. On top of that, getting them switched for analog meters is nearly impossible. If that weren't enough, houses today are jam packed together which means I have to worry about neighbors Wi-Fi and technology use. The only feasible option in that scenario would be to purchase a house, paint it with EMF protection paint, and hope that 5G won't penetrate through. Oh, and let's say I move into that house and a cell tower is installed right next to me, it's not like there's anything I can do about that (there are laws allowing cell towers to go up pretty much wherever they want to and cannot be taken down even if proof is provided that they are emitting unsafe radio frequency levels that are making me sick). I'd then be forced to move. See what I mean? There's no avoiding technology in today's world.

The thought of purchasing land in a remote area is still something I think about but that has its own difficulties. For one, it's expensive. Also, every time I've left my house to go and look for land, I've run into problems as you already know. So, what do I do? Right now, I'm just sticking to my routine and hoping I'll get to a point where I won't be EHS anymore. It would be nice to have a place in this world where me and the millions of other people suffering with EHS could walk outside, go to restaurants, shop in stores, and socialize without the fear and pain associated with EMFs.

Until then, I'll continue to be an EHS Warrior, fighting the invisible enemy, and being the change I want to see. You never know, one day the world may wake up and realize just how bad EMFs really are. Fingers crossed.

My EHS Family

Becoming EHS is one of the best things that happened to me. I know that may sound strange, especially after reading how difficult the journey has been, but it's the truth. For once in my life, I am able to see people for who they are. I am able to connect on levels I never knew existed and I owe it all to my fiancé.

Before her, being EHS was a burden I carried alone. I hid my condition from the world, and hoped it would just disappear. Not only did she show me that having EHS wasn't a burden, but she lightened the load by teaching me it was a gift. Thanks to her, I have been able to reach a large community of people suffering from EHS and passed along the gift of believing them. Something I needed and never received until her.

Many of her patients after hearing my story, related. Although they had stories of their own, they all relatively were the same. I bet you're wondering how I know this and the answer is that I've met them. I've personally gone to numerous of her patients' homes, conducted home EMF inspections and most importantly, I just talked to them. I let them know that they were not alone, just like my girlfriend did for me.

Each person I met, had been through a lot. Some more than me, and for longer. After making the same changes I did in my life, they too are on the road to recovery. For me, I can honestly say that I found what makes me happy in life: being there for other people who are going through difficult times due to the complexity of EHS. I'm proud to say that I have an

EHS family now, growing by the minute, and it's all thanks to my fiancé who was there for me when I had no one.

Chapter 4

Weird Symptoms

Throughout the process of being sick, there were numerous symptoms experienced with little explanations as to "why". These symptoms were unlike anything I had ever experienced and therefore categorized as "weird". Below I have broken them down into sub sections in order to focus on each symptom individually. Some of the symptoms were related to Lyme Disease, some for Mold Illness, but most were in relation to Electromagnetic Hypersensitivity (EHS). Although I may not have all the answers as to why these weird symptoms occurred, my honest attempt at figuring them out is noted.

As far as why these were not included within the original story, there were way too many symptoms and stories that were occurring simultaneously. They are in no particular order and as scary as some of them may be, I can assure you that they are 100% true. Continue reading at your own discretion.

Inflammation

In order to combat the constant inflammation I was suffering from, as well as low testosterone levels, I decided (with approval from my doctor) to try testosterone therapy. From what I was told, testosterone helps reduce inflammation levels within the body and by having levels close to zero, it made sense as to why my body was inflamed.

At first it seemed to work, my head felt better, I had more energy, and my brain fog had lessened. However, I was still having episodes where my heart would suddenly stop or beat erratically. I remember being confused because my inflammation was gone but new symptoms took its place. It was then that I realized a connection. The testosterone was thickening my blood, causing adverse effects in my body and towards my heart. So, I stopped taking it and the symptoms went away. Shortly after stopping testosterone therapy, my inflammation came back, leaving me feeling worse than before.

I then tried alternative methods to get rid of the inflammation. One of which being medical marijuana. After obtaining my medical marijuana card, I experimented with different doses of edible marijuana until I found an amount that took away a lot of my pain. Sadly, that's all it did. I was still experimenting inflammation, so I stopped using medical marijuana and continued my search for an alternative method.

One thing that worked for a short period of time was applying ice to my entire head. This helped reduce the inflammation in my head but was only a temporary solution. Once the ice was removed and my head began warming up, the inflammation would return.

Months later, after living EMF free the inflammation disappeared. It was then that I discovered the correlation to EMFs and inflammation. Whenever I'm around high levels of EMFs, my brain begins to feel inflamed, then my chest, and eventually my entire body. It feels as if I'm submerged deep under water or climbing a really high mountain. After getting out of EMFs, it originally took a few months for the inflammation to vanish. Now, if I'm around high levels of EMFs and begin to feel inflamed, I remove myself from the environment and within hours the inflammation disappears. If I'm around EMFs for a prolonged period of time with no opportunity to avoid them, I'll also take a Tylenol once I am out of the environment in order to aid my body in decreasing the inflammation. Removing myself from EMFs has eliminated my inflammation 100% and only occurs when I am around them.

I have also concluded that there is a connection between low testosterone levels and EMFs.

Throat Problems

I don't remember exactly when my throat problems began, but at one point swallowing became difficult. I no longer had the ability to chug water and would have to hold each sip inside my mouth for up to a minute before being able to swallow. Also, my voice became raspy as if I had been yelling a lot. These symptoms regarding my throat resulted in not wanting to open my mouth to drink water, let alone speak.

My original thoughts were that I had strep throat, but after visiting the doctor and being told that my culture came back negative, I was lost for answers. For months my throat problems remained, leading me to accept that I would have to live with them forever and eventually forgot about them altogether. At some point years later, towards the end of my healing process, my voice became normal and swallowing became easy again.

It wasn't until I exposed myself to high levels of radio frequencies and the symptoms returned, that I noticed a connection. Being around radio frequencies like Wi-Fi, Bluetooth, and cell towers, my voice becomes raspy, I have difficulty swallowing water, my throat becomes sore, and sometimes my throat feels as if it's closing. All of that goes away within a few hours of being away from radio frequencies. On occasion it has taken up to 2 days for my throat to return to normal, all depending on the level of exposure and duration.

Floaters

Prior to getting sick, I had perfect vision. My eyesight was clear, and I had zero "floaters". Let me explain what I mean by floaters. When you look straight ahead at a white wall, these black floating squiggly and sometimes circular objects, move across your field of vision. You can't look directly at them because they float away so you have to use your peripheral vision to look at them. From my understanding, they are within the eye and not something that can be "washed away".

Randomly one day, I had floaters. Although lots of people have them (so I've been told), I never did and the first time I noticed them, they scared me. They almost looked like little worms or spirochetes, so naturally I freaked out thinking I had worms in my eyes.

After finding out that they weren't worms, I felt better but I was still curious as to why they appeared out of nowhere. Over time they progressively got worse and a new eye symptom joined the confusion. On top of the floaters, I now had "twinkling/sparkling dots" that looked like stars in my line of sight. They were subtle but once again, scary.

I asked numerous doctors as well as conducted as much research as I could on "floaters", and yet received no answers as to why they suddenly appeared. The typical answer I received was "everyone has them, they get more visible with age." I didn't accept that answer then, and still don't today. In my defense, how could I possibly go from not having any to eyes filled with them seemingly over night?

What worked for me was blue light blocking glasses. Wearing them all day every day, over time the large amount I once had in my eyes has dwindled down to just a few and the twinkling/sparkling dots only rarely appear. Now I can't say for sure that it was the glasses that made them disappear, but it is a coincidence that in my opinion, merits further investigation.

I have noticed a correlation to the number of floaters I have and the duration of time spent around high levels of EMFs. If I am out of EMFs completely, I have zero floaters. When I am around EMFs, floaters do appear, but there are far less when wearing my blue light blocking glasses. Without them the floaters come back completely, as do the twinkling/sparkling dots.

Red Eyes

Besides floaters, there is one other symptom worth mentioning regarding my eyes. For as long as I can remember, my eyes were dry and red. To counter this, I would carry eye drops with me wherever I went, using them up to ten times a day. At first, I thought it was lack of sleep. Which made sense because at the time I was only sleeping 4-5 hours per night. But even after increasing the amount of sleep I got each night to a minimum of 8 hours, the dryness and redness remained.

After discovering that I had high levels of toxic mold in my body, I correlated the dryness and redness to mold exposure. Yet, after completing multiple mold detoxification protocols, the dryness and redness remained.

Using blue light blocking glasses was another attempt made at eliminating the symptoms. They didn't work though and my eyes still remained dry and red.

Years later, after a few months of living EMF free, my eyes completely cleared up. I thought it was the result of getting healthier and didn't make the connection to EMFs until the symptoms came back again. Learning from my past, I began tracking whenever my eyes would become symptomatic, leading to the conclusion that whenever I am around EMFs my eyes become dry and red. By avoiding EMFs, my eyes are crystal clear.

White Spot

When the vibrations in my body first began, I figured out how to stop them. At the time, what I did was an act of desperation to find relief, and I do not recommend trying it. The vibrations felt similar to a cat purring, only deep within your body and wherever they occurred, pain followed. It almost felt as if my body was falling asleep, similar to the "pins and needles" feeling that would occur upon waking it up. They would begin in my legs and move throughout my body, ending up where I had the greatest blood flow. If I clenched my fist as hard as I could, the vibrations would travel through my body and into my hand. For hours I would sit there, playing with the vibrations by moving them from hand to hand. That was until the vibrations made its way into my head, causing me to faint from the pain.

Upon waking up, I noticed a predominate white spot located on the tip of my nose. It looked strange, was circular in shape, and had a wax type feeling. By moving my finger over the white spot in a similar fashion to a lymphatic massage, I noticed the spot begin to move. It moved from the top of my nose, to under my eye, and then into my temple. From my temple, I massaged it downward toward my neck until it eventually disappeared. Moments later, the vibrations began again in my left foot. The timing was too much of a coincidence for me to ignore, so I took my shoe and sock off to look for any white spots. Sure enough, accompanying the vibrations in my foot was a white spot. It was the exact same shape, same size, and even the same wax texture.

My immediate thought was that it was some sort of parasite, as I watched it travel from my foot up my leg. It traveled slow, as did the vibrations and pain. This is when the act of desperation occurred. I'm not sure why exactly I decided to do what I did next, but I was fearful and didn't want the white spot to travel any further. So, I relaxed my entire body, forced as much blood into my left foot by standing on it, and watched the white spot travel back down into my foot. Once it was inside of my foot, I grabbed a cord and wrapped it tightly around my ankle, cutting off the circulation to my left foot. The vibrations were then only inside of my foot, along with the white spot. For approximately 10 minutes I watched my foot turn red with blood, and witnessed the white spot trying to get past the tightly wrapped cord. After that, my foot began to sweat profusely and was extremely hot to the touch. What concerned me even more, was the smell that was coming from the sweat on my foot. It had sort of a sulfur-like smell and the sweat itself was sticky. I then began thinking that whatever the white spot was, was causing the sweat and foul smell. That led me to my next crazy idea.

I decided to put a Ziplock bag around my foot, and

duct tape it closed, along with the cord that cut off the circulation. That resulted in the bag filling up with steam and sweat. For the rest of that day, I kept the bag secured to my foot and felt the vibrations nowhere else in my body. That was until I had to leave my house for work.

Leaving my house to go to work, I took off the cord as well as the Ziplock bag and to my surprise the vibrations had stopped. Inspecting my foot, I also noticed no white spot and concluded that whatever it was, I sweated it out. That night while at work, the vibrations did not occur a single time. When I arrived back home, I took my shoes and socks off at the front door and noticed the vibrations start again in my left foot. This time though, they were stronger and felt more like a bunch of bees buzzing in my foot, rather than a cat purring. Also, the white spot was back and twice the size. So once again, I grabbed my cord and tried to trap it inside my foot.

For the rest of that night and well into the morning, I was unsuccessful at trapping the white spot inside my foot. I couldn't sleep due to the vibrations coursing through my body and had spent the time researching "traveling white spots" online. After finding nothing on the subject, and the vibrations still occurring, I decided to try and ignore it. That clearly didn't work, and left me feeling scared that I was going to vibrate forever.

The vibrations remained for the rest of the day, until that night when I left the house to run errands. The second I left the house, the vibrations stopped completely. I remember pulling over before getting to the store, and inspecting my body for white spots with a flashlight. There were no white spots or vibrations, which made me think that it was all in my head.

When I arrived back home the vibrations began again, leaving me clueless as to what was going on with my body. The next day I went to the doctors and informed him of the traveling white spot. However, since it only occurred at my house, the doctor had no proof to go off of and thought that it was stress related. I agreed and left his office with his last remark being "if it happens again, take a picture."

After getting home from the doctor's office, the vibrations began again and I immediately took a picture. The white spot was clearly on my left foot within the picture, so I made another appointment with the doctor to bring in my proof. At my next appointment I showed the doctor the white spot and this time he had a look on his face that I was all too familiar with, confusion. He had no clue what it was and after examining my foot he concluded that it could be an allergic reaction to something in my house. This was a relief for me, mainly because someone else believed me but also because I had a possible answer.

I spent the next day washing and cleaning every inch of my house. The vibrations were still there traveling throughout my body, but I ignored them thinking that once my house was clean, they would go away. With my house clean, the vibrations remained. After that, they grew stronger, as did the white spots size. At this point, the white spot was the size of my fist and could be seen moving along my body with the vibrations. It seemed as if the longer I spent within my house, the greater the vibrations became. I then contacted my doctor again, who claimed that he had no answers for me and referred me to a therapist.

I knew I wasn't crazy but after hearing his recommendation to go to a therapist, I lost all hope at getting a cure. For the next few weeks, I ignored the vibrations as they grew and thought they would eventually stop. I took on stress relieving yoga and cut my work load in half. All in an attempt to lower my stress load, as per the doctors' original thought as to why I was experiencing the vibrations. Eventually I grew tired of waiting for it to go away and began experimenting on my body again.

Lying flat on my stomach on my bed and with my left arm hanging over the side, I was able to trap the vibrations by forcing blood into my hand. I used the same cord that I used on my ankle to wrap around the top of my arm and over my shoulder. This cut the circulation off to my entire arm, trapping the vibrations inside. However, rather than my arm turning red with blood, it turned a strange white color. Touching my shoulder resulted in "pitting" and felt extremely clay-like, similar to the wax feeling of the white spot. Eventually I concluded that the white spot had grown and was now the size of my arm.

I then went through the same procedure as I did on my ankle, and wrapped my arm in plastic. The same sticky sweat appeared, as did the sulfur-like smell. After that, I stupidly decided to cut into my shoulder to see if the white spot would drain. Surprisingly, a

In order to avoid feeling that way, I stick to a strict low EMF/body voltage environment.

Bleeding

Random bleeding from my body occurred almost daily for approximately 1 year. It first started with nose bleeds, then from my ears, then in my urine, then in my stool, and ending with my mouth. Although the bleeding eventually stopped, it was definitely one of the scarier symptoms that occurred.

At first, I was experiencing daily nose bleeds, typically in the evenings from 5:00-6:00PM. They occurred no matter where I was or what I was doing and lasted approximately 3 minutes. The fact that they occurred at the same time every day was the only pattern I could find at the time. I had no meters to check EMF levels, no one to ask why they were occurring, and couldn't find any answers while researching. For three full months, the nose bleeds came every single day until one day they randomly stopped. Nothing in my daily routine had changed, my diet was the same, and yet they stopped completely.

When the nose bleeds stopped, bleeding from my ears began. This time though, no pattern occurred. The first time I noticed my ear was bleeding, I mistook it for another nose bleed. It was morning time and my pillow case was covered in blood. The first thing I did was check my nose and to my surprise there was no blood at all. It was confusing. So, I changed my pillowcase, and went into the bathroom to take a shower. While in the bathroom, I looked at myself in the mirror, and noticed no blood near my nose. It wasn't until I hopped in the shower and noticed the water beneath me turning red that I realized the blood was coming from somewhere else. I immediately got out of the shower and checked the mirror again. This time, my beard was red on the side of my face. From what I assume happened, the blood had dried and was hidden in my beard only to be revealed by the water washing it away. Upon further investigation, it became obvious that the blood had come from my right ear.

Once again, I had no one to ask why this was happening and could not find any answers while researching. For months my ears took turns bleeding at night. Sometimes it was my right ear, sometimes my left. There was no pattern as to when it occurred, but only happened while I was asleep. I know this because I stayed up all night on a few separate occasions, and no blood came. The only thing that seemed to help was propping myself up in bed as if I were sitting in a chair and sleeping that way. Lying flat the bleeding always occurred but while propped up the bleeding only happened on a few occasions. After about a month of sleeping (trying to sleep at least) propped up, the bleeding in my ears stopped. The only thing in my daily routine that had changed was sleeping propped up, everything else remained the same.

Once the bleeding in my ears stopped, I soon noticed I was bleeding while I urinated. At first the urine in the toilet was a rust color and my initial thought was that I was dehydrated. So, I upped my water intake in order to hopefully fix the problem. After a few days of rusty urine, my urine soon turned bright red. Seeing blood coming out of me and filling the toilet took my breath away. It was something that had never happened to me before and honestly scared me. The only answers I could find while researching was that my kidneys were damaged but I thought "how could my kidneys be damaged? I don't drink alcohol, and I drink plenty of water." So, I ignored it.

While using the restroom, it didn't burn, it didn't hurt, blood just came out as if it were urine. I had no pain in my abdomen or anywhere else in my body before, during or after urinating. There was no pattern as to when it occurred, and happened almost every other day, once a day. It never happened at the same time, and it didn't matter how much water I was drinking. My urine could be clear all day from drinking water and then randomly it would turn red from blood. Or it would occur first thing in the morning after waking up. This random occurrence of blood in my urine lasted for approximately two months and then stopped. Nothing in my daily routine had changed, minus the fact that I upped my water intake.

When the blood in my urine stopped, I then began noticing blood in my stool. Not only was it in my stool, but it was also on the toilet paper used. The amount of blood coming out was by far the most I had seen up until that point. It was always bright red in color, and poured out of me as if I were urinating from my rectum. From what I learned while researching, I assumed that I had a hemorrhoid and it had burst. Nothing else made sense but once again I had nobody to ask why this was happening, so I ignored it. This occurred for approximately one month and happened every time I passed stool. There was no pattern in regards to time or place, and no matter what I ate or drank it still happened. Then one day, it just stopped.

When the blood in my stool had stopped, randomly I began bleeding from my mouth. At first, I thought it was from brushing my teeth too hard or from not flossing every day. The blood seemed to come from all over my mouth and occurred mainly at night, with no set time frame. It didn't matter if I brushed my teeth or flossed, the bleeding would just start. Each time my mouth started to bleed, it would last for approximately 3 to 5 minutes. It was always bright red in color, never dark and if I smiled, the blood would turn my teeth red. This happened almost every other night for 4 months. I found no reason as to why my mouth was bleeding other than if I were brushing too hard or not flossing enough. After 4 months, the bleeding from my mouth stopped. The only change in my daily routine was that I flossed more regularly and brushed my teeth as gentle as I could while still being effective.

To this day I randomly will still bleed from one of my ears, my mouth will bleed very rarely, and on occasion I will have blood in my stool. However, those symptoms only happen on an extremely rare basis. Bleeding while I urinate hasn't happened since it stopped, nor has bleeding from my nose. I am still unsure as to why I was bleeding from my body in the first place, but I thought it was beneficial to include under weird symptoms.

BRIAN R. HUMRICH

Hot-Colds

Out of all the strange symptoms experienced, this one lasted the shortest amount of time. It began late one night, preventing me from sleeping and would occur in 3 minute intervals. At first, I thought it was the flu, but after figuring out its pattern, I realized it was EMF related. The story of the "hot-colds" began that night.

Lying in bed, a wave of heat hit my body, causing me to sweat through my sheets. The air conditioning was set to 74 degrees and yet I was burning up. My skin was red, my entire body was dripping with sweat, and my breathing became shallow and panicked. But just as sudden as the heat hit me, it went away within a few minutes. Immediately afterwards, I felt as if I were in the snow. My body was ice cold to the touch, my teeth were shivering, and all my joints were locked up in an almost frozen position. Then a few minutes later, the cold left my body and was replaced with the same hot feeling from minutes before.

For about an hour, my body went back and forth from extremely hot to extremely cold, lasting only minutes. The first thing that came to mind was that I had the flu but as the pattern continued from hot to cold, cold to hot, I realized it couldn't be the flu and began searching my home for any other EMF emitting devices thinking it had to be related. For hours I searched, still experiencing the hot-colds, and came up empty handed. My entire home was completely empty of EMFs.

After not finding any EMFs to explain my symptoms, I gave up and got back into bed. That night, I didn't sleep and around 6:00AM, the symptoms stopped. My body temperature normalized and it was as if it never happened. I remember thinking "what was what? Did I have the flu for 8 hours? Did I eat something bad?" However, nothing I thought of could explain the back and forth hot-colds I had experienced.

The rest of that day, my body was normal. No spikes of heat, or drops of cold. Then at around 7:00PM, it started again. This time though, I timed it and tracked my symptoms.

1. **7:01PM-** Hot, nauseas, dizzy, pouring sweat, ringing in ears
2. **7:05PM-** Cold, body aches, skin tightness, cough, shortness of breath
3. **7:08PM-** Hot, nauseas, dizzy, pouring sweat, ringing in ears
4. **7:011PM-** Cold, body aches, skin tightness, cough, shortness of breath
5. **7:014PM-** Hot, nauseas, dizzy, pouring sweat, ringing in ears
6. **7:17PM-** Cold, body aches, skin tightness, cough, shortness of breath
7. **7:21PM-** Hot, nauseas, dizzy, pouring sweat, ringing in ears
8. **7:25PM-** Cold, body aches, skin tightness, cough, shortness of breath
9. **7:28PM-** Hot, nauseas, dizzy, pouring sweat, ringing in ears
10. **7:31PM-** Cold, body aches, skin tightness, cough, shortness of breath
11. **7:34PM-** Hot, nauseas, dizzy, pouring sweat, ringing in ears

12. **7:37PM-** Cold, body aches, skin tightness, cough, shortness of breath
13. **7:40PM-** Hot, nauseas, dizzy, pouring sweat, ringing in ears
14. **7:43PM-** Cold, body aches, skin tightness, cough, shortness of breath
15. **7:47PM-** Hot, nauseas, dizzy, pouring sweat, ringing in ears
16. **7:50PM-** Cold, body aches, skin tightness, cough, shortness of breath
17. **7:53PM-** Hot, nauseas, dizzy, pouring sweat, ringing in ears
18. **7:56PM-** Cold, body aches, skin tightness, cough, shortness of breath
19. **7:59PM-** Hot, nauseas, dizzy, pouring sweat, ringing in ears

This continued until I couldn't take it anymore and decided I'd try and regulate my body temperature with a shower. I started out in the shower with the temperature extremely hot, which counterbalanced the cold I was feeling in my body. Then, when my body switched to being extremely hot, I turned the water to as cold as it would go and that counterbalanced my body's temperature. As long as I stayed in the shower, changing the water temperature to counterbalance my body's temperature, I was fine. That night I took a 4 hour shower.

When the symptoms seemed to subside, I got out of the shower and tried to go to sleep. That didn't happen though. Approximately 10 minutes into trying to fall asleep, the hot feeling hit my body once again. Only this time, I shouted "ARE YOU KIDDING ME?!", causing my girlfriend to wake up. Explaining the symptoms to her was difficult but eventually she understood and had an alternative method for regulating my body temperature.

Her alternative method was called "hydrotherapy", something I had never heard of. She got a towel, soaked it in ice cold water and when my body was in the "hot phase" of the hot-colds, she placed it on my exposed back. Within seconds I would feel better, but the towel would dry up instantly. We even tried putting ice packs on my body, but the ice would melt the second it touched my skin. When the "cold phase" of the hot-colds began, wrapping me up in blankets was the only thing she could think of, so we tried that as well. Eventually I ended up feeling bad that I was keeping her up all night, and went back into the shower to try and regulate my body temperature on my own. At that point it was 3:00AM.

For the rest of that night, I stayed in the shower, regulating my body temperature by using hot and cold water. At around 6:00AM, still in the shower, I fell asleep. Upon waking up minutes later, I realized my body was no longer experiencing the hot-colds and concluded something was going on from 7:00PM-6:00AM causing my body to go through a rollercoaster of temperatures.

For the next several nights at around 7:00PM, the symptoms would begin and rather than complain, I got into the shower. For me, that was the only way I could resolve the problem while still being able to think about the pattern of symptoms I was experiencing. Outside of the shower and experiencing the hot-colds, my brain fog was horrible, but within the shower I could at least think (as well as control my body temperature).

Night after night, I spent approximately 6 hours total within the shower. The other 6-7 hours were spent circulating ice cold towels and ice packs, and wrapping myself up in blankets. Back and forth, every 3 minutes. It was torturous to say the least. For a month, I barely slept.

After that month, I had the idea to pull out my radio frequency meter while I was tracking my symptoms. To my surprise, every 3 minutes the meter would spike, directly correlating with my symptoms. Here's what I had found:

1. **7:00PM-** Hot, nauseas, dizzy, pouring sweat, ringing in ears
    a. **Radio Frequency=** 35 microwatts per meter squared ($\mu W/m2$)
2. **7:03PM-** Cold, body aches, skin tightness, cough, shortness of breath
    a. **Radio Frequency=** 16 $\mu W/m2$
3. **7:06PM-** Hot, nauseas, dizzy, pouring sweat, ringing in ears
    a. **Radio Frequency=** 41 $\mu W/m2$
4. **7:09PM-** Cold, body aches, skin tightness, cough, shortness of breath
    a. **Radio Frequency=** 20 $\mu W/m2$
5. **7:12PM-** Hot, nauseas, dizzy, pouring sweat, ringing in ears
    a. **Radio Frequency=** 38 $\mu W/m2$
6. **7:15PM-** Cold, body aches, skin tightness, cough, shortness of breath
    a. **Radio Frequency=** 18 $\mu W/m2$

7. **7:18PM-** Hot, nauseas, dizzy, pouring sweat, ringing in ears
    a. **Radio Frequency=** 52 µW/m2
8. **7:21PM-** Cold, body aches, skin tightness, cough, shortness of breath
    a. **Radio Frequency=** 29 µW/m2
9. **7:24PM-** Hot, nauseas, dizzy, pouring sweat, ringing in ears
    a. **Radio Frequency=** 33 µW/m2
10. **7:27PM-** Cold, body aches, skin tightness, cough, shortness of breath
    a. **Radio Frequency=** 20 µW/m2
11. **7:30PM-** Hot, nauseas, dizzy, pouring sweat, ringing in ears
    a. **Radio Frequency=** 43 µW/m2
12. **7:34PM-** Cold, body aches, skin tightness, cough, shortness of breath
    a. **Radio Frequency=** 22 µW/m2
13. **7:37PM-** Hot, nauseas, dizzy, pouring sweat, ringing in ears
    a. **Radio Frequency=** 61 µW/m2
14. **7:40PM-** Cold, body aches, skin tightness, cough, shortness of breath
    a. **Radio Frequency=** 50 µW/m2
15. **7:44PM-** Hot, nauseas, dizzy, pouring sweat, ringing in ears
    a. **Radio Frequency=** 35 µW/m2
16. **7:47PM-** Cold, body aches, skin tightness, cough, shortness of breath
    a. **Radio Frequency=** 16 µW/m2
17. **7:50PM-** Hot, nauseas, dizzy, pouring sweat, ringing in ears
    a. **Radio Frequency=** 29 µW/m2

In between the spikes of high radio frequencies, the readings would normalize and stay at around 1 μW/m2. The spikes would last for 10 seconds at the most, then normalize for about 3 minutes dropping down to 1 μW/m2 and then spiking back up again at the end of the 3 minutes. Cycling back and forth every 3 minutes from high readings, to low readings. Just like my symptoms were doing, hot for 3 minutes, cold for 3 minutes.

At 7:00PM each night, the meter would begin spiking and at 6:00AM every morning it would stop. Like clockwork, night after night, it was timed at every 3 minutes all night long. Knowing that my symptoms were correlated with the spikes of high EMFs, I spent the next month driving myself crazy trying to find the source. Some nights the spikes came from my neighbors on the right of me, while other nights it came from my garage area. But always at 3 minute intervals, occurring during the same time frame.

At one point I assumed that it was my smart meter, which pulsed high radio frequencies every 3 minutes. However, that didn't explain why it was only occurring at night, as my smart meter pulsed every 3 minutes even during the day.

Then I began thinking the hot-colds were a reaction to the food that I had been eating. Although my diet was clean, I did sometimes consume salty foods. So, in order to cancel that out, I stopped eating foods that contained high levels of salt. This however, did not fix my problem.

A little while later, my girlfriend bought some flowers at the store and brought them home. They were her favorite, Lilly's. The instant she brought them home, the entire house smelled like flowers and I began to sneeze. She assumed that I was allergic to them and asked if I wanted her to get rid of them. Since I had never been allergic to anything in my life, I told her no and dealt with the sneezing. That night, the hot-colds were worse than they had ever been and once again she assumed that it was the flowers. This time though, rather than ask me if I wanted her to get rid of them, she took them out to the trash and threw them away. That didn't solve anything, as my symptoms remained.

The next day while sitting in my dining room, I began sneezing again. Which caused me to look up at my ceiling and notice the air conditioning vent. The thought that went through my head at that point was that the air coming through the filters must be moldy and that I was reacting to the mold. I then took out my air quality meter and tested the air in my home, just to be sure. The results were in the red, meaning that the air quality was poor. Just to make sure the air quality meter wasn't broken, I tested the air outside in my backyard as well. This showed that the air within my home was worse than the air outside. At that point I thought I had solved my hot-cold problem and decided to change out my air filters. They were black, and smelled extremely bad.

After changing my air filters, the air quality within my home improved and I no longer was sneezing. Sadly, the hot-colds still remained, which made me feel as if I were never going to figure out what was causing them. That night when the hot-colds began, my girlfriend offered me a supplement called "G.I. Detox", which was a binder designed to bind the things in my gut that I was unable to detox. Within 30 minutes, the hot-colds completely stopped and for the first time in months I was able to fall asleep without having to be in the shower all night.

With the G.I. Detox working night after night, my girlfriend made the assumption that I may have had a Candida overgrowth in my gut. Her assumption was based on the knowledge that large doses of IV antibiotics could disrupt gut flora. A stool test was then conducted, proving her assumption correct and revealing that Candida as well as other infections were present. Since I had cut sugar out of my diet, and sugar feeds Candida, she said it was something that could be fixed by completing a round of Candida detox supplements as well as completing more colon hydrotherapies.

While getting my first colon hydrotherapy after starting the Candida detox supplements, I had my first hot-cold experience away from my home and outside of the normal time frame it occurs. Laying on the table, with the speculum inside of me, I felt the hot colds occurring like clockwork every 3 minutes. It was horrible, but at the same time I had a new variable to work with and was somewhat happy. I knew then that it wasn't due to my smart meter, flowers, or mold, and more than likely because of Candida overgrowth.

After completing the Candida detox supplements as well as twice weekly colon hydrotherapies, the hot-colds stopped. Since then I have yet to experience the terrible hot-cold symptoms again and have not had to take prolonged showers in order to regulate my body temperature. I am happy to report that my body remains temperature compliant.

My Penis

One of the most uncomfortable yet important symptoms experienced is in regards to my penis. The reason why I am sharing this with you is because there is very minimal research on the subject and I thought it may help someone else out if I am one of the first to discuss it.

As a man, my penis is of extreme importance and when it no longer worked, I was concerned. I know what you're thinking, erectile dysfunction is common, and it is, but I was 28 years old when this occurred. That, is less common.

Not only did it stop functioning sexually, but it completely retreated inside my body. Worse than any "shrinkage" I had ever experienced; it straight up disappeared inside of me. Each time I had to use the restroom, I literally had to pull it out of me. Awkward, I know.

For years I never spoke about it and figured that's just how it was going to be. I refrained from sex, to avoid feeling uncomfortable or embarrassed, and never really brought it up again. That was until the doctor at the Lyme and Cancer treatment center revealed my extremely low testosterone levels. For some reason I mentioned my inability to achieve an erection and to him it made sense with my low testosterone levels. He prescribed me a natural tincture called "Yohimbe" and promised it would solve my problem. Unfortunately, it didn't, yet whenever he asked about it moving forward, I was embarrassed and lied saying "yep, it's all good."

It wasn't until later on down the road that I connected the dots. This may sound strange, but the entire time my body was protecting itself by retreating my penis. Do you remember the chapter on body voltage earlier on? Well that had a lot to do with my problem. The other factor was EMFs, radio frequencies in particular. By lowering my body voltage to as close to zero millivolts as possible and shielding myself completely from radio frequencies, my penis came back to me. It was definitely a joyous moment.

While covered in EMF protection clothing, a radio frequency blocking blanket, and laying in my grounded bed (the lowest body voltage area in my house), I no longer had an issue with any of my previous problems. I remember thinking to myself "seriously? Why didn't I think of that years ago?"

Today, I no longer have an issue with my penis. However, I have figured out that whenever I am around radio frequencies or my body voltage is too high for too long, my penis retreats. It's like a built in alarm system, telling me that I need to get out of EMFs. If I don't listen to my built in alarm system, it typically takes 1-3 days of 24/7 EMF protection for my penis to come out of hiding and regain full operation.

Muscle Loss

For years leading up to getting sick, I built (in my opinion) the perfect body by working out 7 days a week. I was 6'2" tall, weighed 250-260lbs, and had a body fat percentage in the single digits. From the outside, most people assumed I was a meat head and I was fine with that. I loved being big and there wasn't anything that anyone could say to make me feel otherwise. I felt comfortable when I took my shirt off, and loved the way I looked in the mirror. My body was my ultimate masterpiece.

When I got sick, my body was one of the first things that disappeared. Within a few months, I dropped 55lbs of muscle and lost the desire to workout. My skin was saggy and the muscle that was leftover had an "oatmeal" like texture. Losing all that muscle left me feeling extremely self-conscious. I no longer felt comfortable in my skin, which led to a loss of confidence in my overall self.

For the longest time I had identified myself as the "big guy", and cared a lot about the way I looked on the outside. By looking good externally, I felt good about myself internally. Years later, I learned that's not the way it's supposed to be. It may sound cheesy, but I learned a very valuable lesson from losing all of that muscle. I learned that you need to be happy with who you are on the inside in order to love who you are on the outside. It took me losing my muscle in order to see that I wasn't happy with who I was on the inside.

It wasn't easy, but I eventually learned to accept the things that were out of my control, my muscles being one of the main things. Here's what I've learned:

1. Find happiness in the simple things in life.
2. Cherish the things you can control.
3. Surround yourself with people who accept you for who you are and not what you look like.
4. Love yourself.
5. Superficial things don't matter.
6. Patience.

As far as to why I lost all my muscle, only a few theories come to mind. The first is that EMFs damage muscle tissue, interrupt protein synthesis and effect blood flow. Although that is only a theory, I haven't found any evidence to disprove it.

My other theory is that my body is a lot smarter than I give it credit. Maybe the Lyme bacteria or toxic mold was intertwined inside my muscle and therefore my body eliminated the muscle in order to destroy anything that may have been hiding. However, once again that's just a theory.

Today, I am 210lbs and am happy with what I look like. I may not be the "big guy" I used to be but what I look like on the outside means little in comparison to how I feel about myself. On the inside, I'm the biggest guy I know.

Emotions

Prior to getting sick, I used to be very "emotional". Sad movies made me cry, and scary movies left me checking under my bed before I went to sleep. In life, I led with my heart. It got me into trouble a few times, but I can honestly say that at my core I was a lover, not a fighter. I was in touch with my feelings to say the least. Then I got sick.

Along with my memory, my emotions and ability to feel, disappeared. Simultaneously, my brain and heart had shut down. The things that used to make me happy, no longer interested me and sad movies no longer made me cry. It was as if I were all of a sudden, emotionless and monotone. Let me be clear though, I wasn't depressed nor was I all of a sudden "crazy", I was just sick.

I'll never forget the moment I realized that the world wouldn't understand the difference. I was at a neurotherapy session and my neurotherapist asked me to do a homework assignment for him. He asked me to "go home and try to feel each one of the seven basic emotions." That assignment proved to be impossible for me, which was an eye opener because I used to feel so much. The next day I explained to him that I wasn't able to complete the assignment and he asked for me to explain. I explained that I started with the emotion "happiness" and tried to think of anything that made me happy. The difficult part was that I really didn't know what made me happy and therefore couldn't complete that emotion.

We ended up talking after that about me having to

find what makes me happy. That is when I knew he didn't understand. Prior to getting sick, the gym made me happy. It was my happy place. Anytime I were sad, I would hit the weights and all my troubles would disappear. Being sick, I couldn't work out, so my happy place was taken from me. The sun makes me happy, but I don't feel the actual physical representation of the emotion happiness, get it? The only emotion I didn't have trouble with feeling, was anger. Me being sick, and nobody being there for me, made me angry. However, even that emotion soon disappeared, leaving me completely monotone in my feelings.

At that point, I was aware of what emotions were, but felt absolutely nothing. Telling people that though, always ended in me looking crazy. So, I kept it to myself and learned how to avoid situations where emotions were involved. In the beginning this was hard, but after a few years I got good. I learned how to laugh when others laughed, smile when others were happy, and even became an expert at hiding the pain from my symptoms. From the outside, I appeared normal to everyone else, but on the inside I was a wreck.

I'm not proud of having to lie about my emotions, but it's what needed to be done. I learned very early on that not everyone can handle the truth and therefore, hiding it was easier. For a very long time, I hid from the world in order to not appear crazy.

Now, I don't hide. I got rid of the people in my life who made me feel crazy, and now I'm open and honest about the fact that I struggle with emotions.

Mainly because I found a direct link to EMFs. Around EMFs I'm emotionless, but EMF free, I have periods of time where I feel everything. Sometimes it's a little much to handle (sorry, babe) but now I know why I became emotionless, EMF exposure. It's hard to think that EMFs took everything from me, but it's true. Hopefully after enough time of being EMF free, I'll get back to my old emotional self. Until then, at least I have someone in my life who sees through what EMFs have done to me and is in love with who I am at my core.

Sensitivity to Light

One of my first symptoms was a sensitivity to light. Not sunlight, but indoor lighting like fluorescent light bulbs and light from various screens and monitors. Being indoors with the lights on made my head feel like it was going to explode, my eyes felt hot and swollen, and I felt dizzy which made walking tricky. Sometimes standing under a light even for a moment, would make my skin feel like it was burning.

For years I thought it was all in my head, thanks to the people in my life telling me so. It wasn't until a naturopathic doctor informed me that a sensitivity to light was common with toxic mold exposure (which I had), that I stopped thinking it was all in my head. However, even after detoxing my body from mold, the sensitivity to light remained.

The only explanation I could find other than mold exposure, was related to EMFs. Under the category of EMFs was a subject called "dirty electricity". I learned that fluorescent light bulbs create dirty electricity by turning on and off thousands of time per second. The dirty electricity created is detrimental to your health and numerous studies have proven it. Also, the light itself is blue, and blue light suppresses melatonin production. Yet, they are still in use. Recommendations in these studies suggested switching back to incandescent light bulbs, which are difficult to find anywhere other than online.

I tried switching out my light bulbs but even those proved to be too much for me to handle. This resulted in me not using indoor lighting at all, and using candles at night when needed. Today, I still feel the lights above me when I go to the store but because that's my only exposure to fluorescent lights, it's manageable.

Hair Loss

In the past, my hair had always been something I cherished. Getting sick, made my hair start to fall out. Each time I brushed my hair, large chunks would appear in my comb. In the shower, my hair would fall out while scrubbing my head even if I were gentle. No matter what I did, my hair just kept falling out. Most of the people I consulted with this issue would typically shrug their shoulders and say "sucks to get old".

I, however, didn't accept that my age had anything to do with the fact that my hair was falling out. Besides, I had time to figure out why my hair was falling out because I wore an EMF proof hat and could conceal my hair loss from the world.

After a few years of wearing EMF protection on my head 24/7, my hair slowly stopped falling out. Even the hair that had fallen out in chunks grew back. The fact that I never found an answer as to why this was occurring, has stumped me. Somehow, I feel as if there is a link to EMFs and have continued to wear EMF protection on my head 24/7. This has prevented any new hair loss from occurring and I'm happy to report that my hair is almost back to its original state. Too bad the world will never see it though; it's always covered with an EMF protection hat.

Metal

When I first discovered this symptom, it baffled me. Metal, of all things, became somewhat of an allergy for me early on. At least that's what I thought it was, an allergy. Anything metal that I touched, started a chain reaction of vibrations, starting at the source and making its way up my arm.

Simple things like my belt buckle and even door knobs in my house set off my symptoms with a single touch. In the beginning, I tried rationalizing the sudden vibrations by telling myself that I was crazy and that nobody was allergic to metal. I searched endlessly for answers by typing in searches for " sudden allergy to metal" and always came up empty handed.

So, I did what I thought was best and chose to keep it to myself. Secretly though, I avoided all metal, all the time. I switched out my metal latched belt for a non-metal belt. I chose clothing that didn't have any metal on them. I placed tennis balls on my door knobs. I avoided walking on top of manholes and even avoided sitting in metal chairs. All of that was to prevent the vibrations from occurring.

After a very long time of living metal free, I stumbled across a link between EMFs and metal. Somewhere in a book I read, it stated that metal acts as an antenna for EMFs and can amplify signals. It was in that moment that I connected the dots and realized that it wasn't an allergy, but a reaction to the metal acting as an antenna for EMFs.

It all made sense after that. Moving forward I would have to avoid metal that was potentially picking up EMFs. By doing so, my body was able to recover faster. However, avoiding metal was not as easy as it sounds.

There's metal literally everywhere, from the utensils that you use, to the handle in your shower. There's no escaping it.

Today, I still get vibrations up my arm and body when I touch metal, but by following a strict no metal lifestyle, it's manageable.

Tinnitus

Tinnitus is generally defined as a loud pitched ringing in one or both ears. Most would agree that it is annoying and tends to get worse in silence. Night time can be quite challenging as well. For me, it started the moment I became sick.

Every night while trying to fall asleep with the many

symptoms I was experiencing, tinnitus was one that stood out. Researching what caused it always left me more confused. The causes listed didn't apply to me. For example: I don't listen to loud music, so temporary hearing damage was not the answer I was looking for.

After a while, I stopped looking for answers and figured I'd join the large amount of our society who suffer from this mysterious ailment. Luckily, I change my mind a lot and randomly decided one day that I was going to figure out how to stop my tinnitus. This is where the fun began.

In the past, my dad had given me a pair of noise cancelling headphones that he would use at the gun range and were something that I had used to attempt to drown out the ringing. As you already know, silence makes it worse so the noise cancelling headphones weren't sufficient by themselves. The idea to wrap them in faraday tape was a bit of a mystery, but it came to me, so I went with it.

After completely wrapping the headphones in faraday tape and padding the interior with faraday cloth, I tried them on. Once on, the tinnitus was still there, but a strange sensation of my ears "draining" occurred. It felt like I had gone swimming and my ears were releasing the water from the pool. Only, I didn't go swimming, so the sensation was weird.

For the first few days, I wore the headphones everywhere in my house. The draining would occur at random times, and the tinnitus was still there. Being frustrated that the tinnitus was still there, I stepped up my headphone use and wore them at night while I slept as well.

After about a week, I noticed a significant difference in the ringing and knew I was onto something. So many thoughts raced through my head. I remember thinking "there's a connection to EMFs, I know it." That's when I began researching tinnitus and its overwhelming link to EMFs. Shockingly, there are numerous studies on the association, but no real answers on how to cure it.

So, I stuck with my faraday wrapped headphones and hoped for the best. My assumption was that if EMFs caused damage to my inner ear, which led to tinnitus, then blocking my ears as much as possible with my headphones would allow them to heal. I was right.

After a few months of using the headphones at least 12 hours a day, my tinnitus disappeared. On occasion, I still get random high pitched ringing in my left ear, but nowhere near as bad as it once was. When I wear my headphones at night, the only sound I hear is my heartbeat. With the headphones on, I have zero symptoms related to tinnitus. Also, the draining feeling happens on occasion but typically only after a high EMF exposure. When it does occur, I step my headphone wearing up even more and try to let my inner ear heal. If there's one thing this whole process has taught me, it's that time away from EMFs is crucial for the healing process to occur.

Pooling

The most consistently "strange" symptom I experienced was pooling. It happened all day and at night it prevented me from sleeping in any position other than propped up as if I were sitting. Sleeping that way was nearly impossible, but it prevented the pooling sensation from reaching my head. In order to better understand what I was experiencing, let me explain it in basic terms.

It felt as if my body was half filled with some sort of thick liquid. This liquid, depending on what I was doing, would move throughout my body. If I were standing, it would fall to my calves and feet, making them swell and feel heavier than normal. If I were laying down, the liquid would fall into my back, butt, and lower half of my legs. If I were laying down too long, it would make its way to my head and cause a painful heavy feeling. Laying on my left side, the liquid fills up my left and leaves my right side feeling light and empty. If I were laying down and stood up too quickly, the liquid falls to my feet and I get light headed. I even passed out on occasion from standing up too quickly. The liquid within me can be felt slowly moving, as if it were warm water running down the inside of my body.

From what I've gathered, I think the liquid has something to do with either my blood, or my lymphatic fluid. Researching this symptom is nearly impossible, and therefore my explanation is merely a theory. I am unsure as to what this symptom is, but I have figured out how to prevent it.

Avoiding EMFs, once again, results in less pooling. The longer I avoid EMFs, the less my body pools. There are even days where I don't pool at all.

Episodes

Having Lyme disease, I learned about a certain behavior called "Lyme rage". This is a term that may or may not resonate with you. For me, it was something I experienced quite often but never realized the correlation to EMFs until I stopped calling it Lyme rage.

Each and every time I'm around too many EMFs (Wi-Fi, Bluetooth, etc.) for a prolonged period of time, I lose the ability to think. My mind literally goes blank and the only thing I'm even remotely able to focus on, is how bad the pain is.

In those moments, I also seem to get extremely angry and agitated. I have learned how to spot when this is about to happen and have called them "episodes" rather than Lyme rage because in my opinion/personal experience and research, it has nothing to do with Lyme.

An episode typically goes like this:

I start out feeling "normal" with very little symptoms and my health percentage around 80%. Then I leave my house and head to the store for groceries or for an appointment (I usually don't have any other reason to leave). Learning from my past mistakes, I always try to go out at times where the crowds are minimal. Which means I'm leaving the house early in the morning or late at night.

Once out, I pass by cell towers approximately every 30 seconds, and my symptoms begin flaring up. First, my heart starts to race and beat erratically. Then, my head starts to throb. Lastly, my ability to think about anything other than driving disappears and my eyes start to get red.

Cell towers aren't the only thing that cause my symptoms to flair. I also pass by hundreds of homes which are connected to Wi-Fi, have smart meters blasting outwards, and even stop at red lights where the drivers surrounding me are all on their cell phones. Within minutes of leaving my house, I feel trapped in a sea of EMFs.

After about 10 minutes of being out and around that many EMFs, my health percentage drops to around 50%.

Unfortunately, my trips to the store or appointments last longer than 10 minutes so what you've read so far is only the beginning stages of an episode.

Anxiety usually kicks in around the 30 minute mark. This type of anxiety however, is never rational. I know in those moments that I have no reason to feel anxious, but for some reason EMFs trigger something in my body to make me feel that way.

Finding a store that doesn't have a cell tower on it or near it has become harder and harder. All of my previous "safe stores" are now equipped with cell towers on their roofs, so I've had to find alternatives. That however, does not contribute to my anxiety. Weird, I know. The anxiety I feel during the onset of an episode is for no specific reason, other than being in the presence of too many EMFs for longer than my body can handle.

Once I'm inside a safe store, the crowds are minimal but the people shopping are always on their cell phones. Not to mention the plethora of wireless radio frequency cameras, fluorescent lights, and cash registers filling the store. I always come prepared though, with a list of what I need because my mind stops working completely once I step inside the store.

Shortly after leaving the store with my groceries, the anxiety I once had turns to anger. Timeline wise, I'd say this occurs at about the 1 hour mark. The symptoms I experience at this point are: full body vibrations, aches in all of my joints, my muscles feel like they are melting off the bone, my head feels like my brain is swollen and pushing on the inside of my skull, my eyes are bloodshot, and my ability to rationalize disappears. I know I shouldn't be driving in these moments, but my inability to think takes over and all I can focus on is getting home.

The episode has begun. If my girlfriend is with me, I always snap at her. If not, I yell at my steering wheel. Once again, I have no reason to be angry, but this is what EMFs do to me. They change me into a different person. Sort of like the Incredible Hulk. The only difference is, I don't turn green, I turn red. My face tends to look like I had spent the day in the sun.

Depending on how long my exposures are, dictates how bad of an episode it is. More exposure equals a worse episode.

The episode itself consists of random bursts of anger with no explanation as to why I'm angry, and long moments of silence in between. In these times, my health percentage is always around 10%.

Nothing works to calm me down while in an episode, other than removing myself from EMFs as much as possible. As soon as I am out of EMFs, my anger vanishes and my symptoms slowly start to disappear. It usually takes around 30/45 minutes depending on the length of exposure for me to get back to "normal".

It wasn't until a pattern emerged that I noticed a correlation between episodes and EMFs. There is a direct link between the two. So, whenever I start to feel myself getting to the point of an episode, I check my surroundings for any visible sources of EMFs and if I see anything, I immediately remove myself from the situation. Sadly, there are EMFs everywhere, so in order to avoid an episode I tend not to leave my house unless absolutely necessary.

Living this way is difficult but it's necessary if I want to avoid an episode.

On a side note, my record for leaving the house and being around EMFs without an episode is 2 hours.

BRIAN R. HUMRICH

Weather

One of my earliest "strange symptoms" was a reaction to shifts in the weather. This reaction was eventually tied to the weather, but early on was a completely different story.

There are some individuals who I have met that get "itchy knees" or a "strange tingling sensation" in their body prior to it raining. Their symptoms pop up hours before the rain comes, and sometimes even a full day in advance. Other individuals I've met, can literally smell the rain right before it comes.

With me, I felt nothing but pain. The pain would come on approximately 12 hours prior to the weather change, and would increase the closer it got to the actual change. My entire body would feel like it were in a vice, my head felt like it were going to explode, my eyes felt like they were going to pop, my stomach felt like it was being stabbed with a thousand knives, and my tinnitus turned into a "nails on a chalkboard" screeching sound.

Everything I researched on these strange symptoms came back inconclusive. Some articles said it was because of mold in my body, and others said it was normal for people to sense weather changes.

The worst part is that there was nothing I could do in those moments to lessen the pain. I tried everything from: covering my entire body is tinfoil, covering my entire body in faraday cloth, getting inside my faraday tent, taking detox baths, taking supplements to bind whatever was happening inside my stomach, and even tried ignoring it a few times. Nothing worked. It was one of those things that in my opinion, went away with time.

As time moved forward, and I got better, the symptoms related to changes in weather have lessened. However, I still feel "off" when it rains.

Additional thoughts I've had about what other possible reasons I could be experiencing symptoms during weather changes: Barometric pressure, humidity levels, and radio frequencies getting distorted while traveling through rain.

Tile

If you have a difficult time finding your keys, this small plastic device called a "tile" supposedly helps you find them. They're extremely small, but sure do pack a heavy punch when it comes to EMFs. The story I'm about to tell you involves a major miscommunication on my behalf but it's important to tell.

Shortly after starting dating, my girlfriend and I moved in together. Every day she would get up around 5:00am, do her morning routine, and then kiss me goodbye as she left for work. While she and all my neighbors were at work, my body would get an EMF break.

Every day when she would get home, typically around 6:00pm, my symptoms would start up again. Headaches, brain fog, muscle weakness, random twitching, fainting, blurry vision and more, all popped up the second she walked through the door.

At first (and for a long time), I associated this with her. I thought it was her "negative energy" and on numerous occasions accused her of being in a negative mood. She would always counter my accusations with "but babe, I'm in a great mood." This back and forth altercation occurred every day when she got home. Honestly, don't lie, what would you think?

As far as the negative energy goes, let me explain what I meant. Have you ever walked into a crowded room of your friends or colleagues, only for them to stop talking right as you step inside the room? Try to imagine for a second what that feels like. Can you feel the "energy" of the people in the room? Were they talking about you? How do you know? It's a feeling, right? Well that's how I am. I get "vibes" from people and can pick up on their energy from time to time. That's what I thought was happening with my girlfriend. I thought she was in a bad mood or had a bad day at work each time she came through the door. I was sooooo wrong and it pains me deeply to know I made that wrong assumption in regards to her "energy".

The way I figured out it wasn't her energy was by chance. One night, while having debilitating symptoms, I grabbed my radio frequency meter and started scanning my room for the source. This time was different though. This time, it felt like that same "negative energy" I felt when my girlfriend would come home from work. In that moment, I also thought it was her energy but as you'll soon find out, I was wrong then too.

The radio frequency meter was reading so high that it was maxed out, but it came in waves. It would pick up the max reading, then slowly drop down to levels I could stand. The pulsing of the frequencies correlated with the timing of my symptoms so I knew at that point it wasn't my girlfriend's energy. Looking back, it sounds silly that I even thought that, but hey, I'm being honest here.

Anyways, the reading was coming from my girlfriends' purse. Her eyes and mine both lit up when we found the source but we remained confused because it was a purse, and how could a purse put off radio frequencies? I'll never forget what happened next, she grabs her purse, looks over at me, and goes "could this be it?" She held up her keys, and dangling from them was a small plastic device, called a tile. The meter went off like never before. We were both shocked in that moment.

Immediately I grabbed tinfoil and wrapped the device tightly inside a piece. Instantly, the meter reading dropped and my symptoms disappeared. Up until that point, my girlfriend had only heard of me using tinfoil as a way to block radio frequencies, and now she saw it in action. It blew her mind as I remember saying "see, I told you tinfoil worked." However, that's not the end of that story.

Shortly after wrapping the device in tinfoil, we went around the house with the radio frequency meter searching for any other devices that may have been doing the same thing. Due to the fact that we wrongly assumed that because her phone was off, her device wouldn't work, we wanted to see if any other devices were doing the same.

We found one other device, my Bluetooth speaker inside our hall closet that hadn't been used in a long time. It was doing the exact same thing the tile was doing. So, we wrapped that in tinfoil and once again, the meter dropped to acceptable levels, and any remaining symptoms I had, subsided.

It was in that moment that I realized I made a huge mistake. I began putting the pieces together of my girlfriends "negative energy" and her keys with the device on it. That whole time I thought it was her negative energy, but it was actually her keys that I was picking up on. Each time she walked through the door, she had her purse over her shoulder and her keys were inside, sending high pulsed radio frequencies toward my direction.

After explaining to her what I thought, she was relieved that it wasn't her energy that was negative and we both had a good laugh. To this day, when she gets home from work, there hasn't been a single time where I made that mistake again. For those of you who didn't get the mistake I made, let me be clear: I thought that my girlfriend had negative energy, when in reality it was her tile on her keys sending out high radio frequencies. Since I could feel them coming from her direction, I made the assumption that it was her and never thought that it could be something she had in her purse. I was wrong and have done my best to not make mistakes like that again.

Heart Attacks

One of the major symptoms I haven't discussed yet, involves my heart. Around certain EMF technology, my heart acts erratic. It beats fast, then slow, then skips a few beats and sometimes completely stops. Prior to figuring out what it actually was, I thought I was having heart attacks.

The story of how I figured out it was not a heart attack, involves my need for figuring out the "why" behind everything. It's a gift and a curse to have this type of mind. Rather than accept that I was having heart attacks, I wanted to know why it was happening.

My first encounter with what I thought was a heart attack, happened late one night after I had already fallen asleep. Up until this point, my heart on occasion would randomly beat "weird". This night was different.

All of a sudden, I was awoken by the feeling of my heart stopping. I remember not being able to breathe, my heart not beating, and being absolutely terrified. I had never experienced anything like it before and therefore, I thought I was dying. It may have seemed like an overreaction, but when you feel your heart stop, nothing else makes sense.

In that moment, I stood up out of my bed and tried to move around in an attempt to circulate my blood. It was all that I could think of doing, besides give up and let myself die. After about 5 seconds of feeling no beat, my heart thumped extremely hard and began beating again. Thinking it was a one-time thing, I got back into bed and tried to go back to sleep.

Immediately upon laying down, it felt as if my blood was acting weird and moving slower than normal. Seconds later, my heart stopped again. This time, it made a loud thump first, and then stopped. Then it quickly started beating again but in a slower rate than I was used to. I grabbed my pulse oximeter and quickly checked my SpO2 and pulse rate. My heart rate was at 39 beats per minute and my SpO2 was at 79%. Seeing those extremely low numbers terrified me to the point of waking up my girlfriend next to me.

In that moment, my girlfriend was more terrified than I was. Her response to my condition was to take me to the hospital. However, I knew that going to a hospital would only increase my exposure and ultimately my symptoms as well. With the hospital not being an option and her concern for me growing, I told her to go back to sleep and that I would take care of myself. A stubborn remark from a stubborn man, I know.

With her refusing to go back to sleep, I hopped in the shower hoping that my heart problems would disappear. For the next hour I sat in the bathtub with the shower hitting my legs, and she sat on the floor next to me monitoring my condition. I eventually told her that I felt better, even though I didn't, and we both got into bed. After about 10 minutes of her struggling to stay awake, she fell asleep and I was left to deal with my symptoms on my own. I remember thinking that I was glad she fell asleep because I didn't want to worry her. That night, I couldn't sleep. I was too afraid that if I fell asleep, I wouldn't wake up.

Once my girlfriend left for work in the morning, my symptoms disappeared leaving me with the ability to sleep. I slept for a majority of that day and didn't feel any heart related symptoms. At around 5:00pm my girlfriend arrived home and I informed her of the good news " no heart problems all day". She was shocked and we both concluded that it could have been related to a supplement I was taking called "G.I. Detox". We thought that somehow it was doing something negative in relation to my heart and therefore I stopped taking it. The next few nights, I continued to feel as if I were having heart attacks even though I was no longer taking the supplement. With my heart problems still occurring, she continued to insist that I go to the hospital and I continued to insist that I didn't want to go. I was dead-set on figuring out what was wrong with my heart on my own and not get told I was crazy by doctors who were uninformed on EHS.

That night I figured out what was causing my heart problems by chance and learned a very valuable lesson in the process. For some reason I decided to recheck all of the EMF emitting devices within my home, just to double check. The results were shocking. I found one device downstairs, directly underneath where I slept, that was emitting radio frequency levels in the thousands. It was my girlfriends' phone. Her phone was on airplane mode and yet the Bluetooth had somehow come on without her knowledge. Turning off the Bluetooth however, the phone was still emitting extremely large pulses of radio frequencies. Witnessing this, my girlfriend asked "I thought when my phones on airplane mode it doesn't give off any EMFs?" We both were confused, as I had thought the same. We checked my phone for comparison and with it on airplane mode it gave off zero radio frequencies. Her phone though measured over 1,500 µW/m2 while on airplane mode. It was a discovery that confused us both.

Turning her phone off completely was the only thing that seemed to work. Airplane mode was no longer a safe option for her. We spent the next few minutes discussing anything that she had downloaded recently or any updates that could have caused her phone to emit high levels of radio frequencies even while on airplane mode. The only thing she had downloaded was an additional app, which even after deleting it, her phone still acted the same. That night my heart problems were completely absent. I felt absolutely fine and no longer was afraid to fall asleep.

The next day my girlfriend took my radio frequency meter with her to work and tested her phone on and off of airplane mode. She deleted a majority of her apps and retested after removing each one. Nothing worked for her, and her phone remained pulsing high levels of radio frequencies even on airplane mode. After about a week of her keeping her phone off while at home, she grew angry that her phone continued to act up while on airplane mode. At that point she came up with the idea to wipe her phone and restore it back to its factory setting. After that, her phone stopped emitting radio frequencies while on airplane mode.

To this day, we continue to check both of our phones with the radio frequency meter to ensure that they are not pulsing while on airplane mode. There have been a few incidents where her phone continued to pulse while on airplane mode, which was solved by her turning it off completely and turning it back on. This has also been the case for a few other individuals' phones that I have checked while on airplane mode. The lesson I learned is that airplane mode doesn't always work and therefore the safest bet is to just turn your phone off when not in use. With that being said, I no longer experience problems related to my heart as long as I continue to avoid EMFs.

Fingernails and Toenails

Over time as my body healed, I began noticing something strange occurring with my fingernails and toenails. What I noticed was that the majority of my nails were a brownish yellow color, covering the top 75% of each individual nail. On top of the discoloration, they appeared to have strange ridges and varying thickness. The bottom 25% was clear and had a smooth even texture.

Being unsure as to what had caused the discoloration and uneven texture of my nails, I began documenting my new discovery. Every two weeks when I would cut my nails, I would notice the discoloration growing less and less while the new nail grew upward. After about 3 months my nails were at 50% discolored and 50% clear. It looked as if I had painted my nails a brownish yellow color and had let them grow out, revealing an unpainted nail towards the bottom.

During that time, I researched as much as I could on the topic of nail discoloration and found nothing that made sense. The answers found were all in relation to some sort of nail fungus, but that was not what was occurring in my opinion. In the past I had had athletes' foot but never anything that caused the actual nail to change color. Also, the same discoloration was occurring in my fingernails, which led me to believe it wasn't a fungus. In my opinion, the discoloration was due to the state of health my body was in and as I became healthier, so did my nails.

Research also revealed there was no link to Lyme disease, mold illness, or EHS. However, I believe that having all three of those major illnesses caused major damage to my body, which could have contributed to the overall health and discoloration of my nails. Today, my fingernails are completely clear but the strange ridges still cover approximately 25% of the top portions of my nails, growing outward. Rubbing my finger over them there is a clear difference in ridge pattern as well as overall thickness. My guess is that as I continue to regain my health, my fingernails will eventually become normal again. My toenails are another story. They are still 25% discolored and still have observable differences in the ridges as well as the overall thickness. I am unsure as to why my toenails are taking longer to regain clearness, but I assume it has to do with my overall health. Over time I believe my fingernails and toenails will regain their clear color and even thickness as I continue to get healthier.

Metallic Taste

There was a point when one of my symptoms made me feel a little insane. It started while I was driving and drinking from a red bull can. My energy at the time was extremely low and I relied heavily on the use of energy drinks to get me through the day. Upon drinking from the can, I remember the liquid leaving a metallic taste inside my mouth. At least that's what I thought it was from. That night I noticed the metallic taste again in my mouth, but this time while drinking from a plastic water bottle. The fact that I was tasting metal, concerned me enough to bring up the phenomenon with my family, leaving them to think I was even crazier than before.

Discussing weird symptoms with anyone other than my journal became the new norm, as I learned that people judge what they don't understand. The metallic taste in my mouth became an everyday occurrence after that, and would be present even if I weren't drinking any liquids or using anything metal. Looking up this symptom, I was left with no answers that pertained to me and thought that I was going insane. How could a metal taste be present in my mouth if I weren't drinking from anything metal? It was a question that confused me for an extremely long time. Eventually my question was answered by a doctor who claimed that a metallic taste in the mouth is common with individuals experiencing mold illness. That however didn't answer "why" it occurred in the first place and left me searching for answers on my own.

From there I was able to narrow down my search results to "mold illness and metallic taste in mouth" and found numerous individuals experiencing the same weird symptom. None of which though, could explain why this occurred as a result of mold illness. For the next few years the metallic taste would come and go, but one thing remained constant, my lack of taste in general. Foods no longer tasted like they had in the past, and lacked the flavorful smells they once had. It was at that point that I assumed a correlation between mold illness and taste/smell senses being abnormal. This wasn't just in regards to food though. I noticed that mostly everything that once contained a dominant smell in my life became odorless and all liquids lost their taste. It was as if I no longer had the ability to taste or smell anything, but periodically I would however have a random metallic taste in my mouth.

After completing numerous mold detoxification protocols, my sense of smell and taste returned, and the random metallic taste in my mouth hasn't occurred in years. I am still unsure as to why mold illness caused my body's senses to shut down for a period of time, leaving a metallic taste in its place, but I do fully intend on figuring that out in the near future.

Inability to Sweat

The first time I noticed I wasn't sweating presented itself as more of a challenge than a symptom. I was on a walk around my neighborhood, which consisted of numerous hills, and half way through I wasn't sweating. Instead I was left with an overwhelmingly itchy feeling in the locations where I typically would sweat: forehead, chest, back, and armpits. After noticing the lack of sweat, I stepped up my pace and walked faster. At the end of the walk with sweat still not present on my body, it became a goal of mine to figure something that would make me sweat.

At this point I wasn't thinking that it was related to my illness because I was still in the earliest stages of mold, Lyme, and EHS. Instead, I thought it was related to my body having adapted to the pace of the workouts I was doing and therefore a change needed to be made. Instead of going on walks outside, I stepped it up to walking on a treadmill at a gym. After 4 hours of walking and no sweat dripping whatsoever, I began running. That still didn't work. I spent the next few weeks trying to run the sweat out of me and was unsuccessful.

Sometime after trying to use exercise as a means to sweat, I stopped being able to attend the gym as the environment was too much for my illness. That is when I figured out a correlation between my inability to sweat and my illness. Since my body was unable to detox, and sweating is a form of detoxification, it meant that sweating wasn't going to happen. That didn't stop me from trying though. In a desperate attempt to sweat, I purchased an at home portable sauna. It was small, folded up for easy storage, and claimed to be low in EMF. Sitting in the sauna for the first time, I remember expecting to sweat profusely. However, that's not what happened. Instead, I sat there for an hour, itchy in all the spots where I would typically sweat, and turned beat red from the heat. For months I tried to sweat using the sauna but was unsuccessful.

Years later I was so used to not being able to feel the

heat, that it startled me when a bead of sweat dripped down my face. I was walking into my kitchen when it happened and was so confused that I initially thought my house had sprung a leak. When I touched my face to feel what it was, a new drop replaced the one I wiped away within seconds. At that point I knew I was sweating and grew so excited that I shouted "I'm sweating!" It was a very intense moment for me because I knew that my body was reaching a healthier level.

Today, I continue to sweat when sweating is necessary. In my opinion, I stopped being able to sweat because of my body's detoxification pathways being in poor condition and once they were up and running again, my body was able to detox and sweat again. This could have been a combination of the mold illness, Lyme disease, and EHS but I couldn't say which one in particular. Therefore, I am sticking with my theory that it was a result of a poor detoxification system. Moving forward, if I ever stop sweating again, I will know that I need to detox my body.

Random Rashes

When I first found out that I had Lyme Disease, one of the questions I was asked was "Did you have a bullseye rash?" This was asked because individuals who are bitten by a tick carrying the disease will typically leave behind a rash in the shape of a bullseye. However, that was not the case for me. I didn't remember being bitten let alone a rash of any sort. After that is when I started documenting any random rashes I would get, in hopes to provide any connection to what was wrong with my health.

The first random rash was located on my wrists. It was red, scaly, and lasted for approximately 2 weeks. It also itched extremely bad and would not stop itching no matter what creams or ointments I rubbed onto it. The doctor I showed it to said that it looked like a Candida rash and that if I left it alone it would clear up. That wasn't a good enough answer for me, but I left it alone anyways and eventually it did clear up.

Next I noticed the same rash appear on my forearms, only this time it didn't itch at all. It almost looked like I had acne on my forearms, due to the little bumps popping up all over. These lasted for about a week and then randomly disappeared. Once again, my doctor said that it was Candida and that it would go away with time.

After that the rash seemed to jump from my arms and onto my groin region. The rash itself was the same as before, but covered my entire groin as well as my rear end. That is when my doctor confirmed once again that it was definitely Candida. However, he did absolutely nothing to fix the issue or explain how it was happening in the first place. Not to mention that it was a rash that was moving all over the place. That is when I began researching rashes and Lyme Disease and discovered that some people have random rashes that occur well after their original diagnosis. That seemed to be the answer that I was looking for because after that I stopped looking.

A few months later the rash re appeared on my wrists. Then a few weeks later it popped back up on my forearms, then my groin and rear end. It was a cycle that repeated itself over and over again for a few years until eventually I figured out a solution. Avoid EMFs. The longer I have gone without exposing myself to EMFs, the longer I have gone without seeing any random rashes. I'm not sure if they were occurring because of the EMFs I was surrounded by, or as a result of my body trying to detox and pushing out toxins in the only places it was capable of. Either way, I no longer experience random rashes to this day.

Detox Period

After removing as many EMFs as possible from my environment as well as avoiding them to the best of my ability, I noticed my body going through somewhat of a "detox period". For approximately 2 weeks I experienced symptoms unlike my original EHS related symptoms. It began with a slight headache that gradually turned into a migraine, then increased irritability, extreme nausea, and flu like symptoms.

After about 2 weeks, the symptoms disappeared. However, that's not why I came to the conclusion that it was an EMF detox. I came to the conclusion after visiting my parents' house. Their house was EMF central and regardless of the fact that I was EHS, they did nothing to reduce the levels when I came over.

Arriving at my parents' house the first thing I noticed was the plethora of wireless security cameras covering the front entrances putting off levels of radio frequencies exceeding 1,000 μW/m2. At the front door there was a wireless "ring" security doorbell that put off well over 2,000 μW/m2. Once inside, they had multiple wireless Wi-Fi routers as well as a range extender, each putting off radio frequency levels higher than my meter could measure. On top of that, they had numerous "smart" televisions throughout the home, each measuring 150 μW/m2 when off, and well over 2,000 μW/m2 when on. The rest of their home contained numerous Bluetooth devices, iPads, computers, and a wireless sensor for the new pool they installed. Those readings created a fog of EMFs blanketing the air with readings ranging from 100 μW/m2 to over 2,000 μW/m2. In their backyard, more security cameras were present, measuring around 1,000 μW/m2 standing beneath them. The worst part about being in their home was the fact that they refuse to turn any of the above mentioned devices off while I'm around, even if it meant I'd be in pain. On occasion however, my mom has turned her phone on airplane mode.

Arriving at their home was like walking into a war zone. The background constant radio frequency levels within their home never dropped below 1,800 μW/m2, no matter where I was. Explaining this to them was something that always resulted in foul looks, and disagreeing remarks. To them, EHS was in my head, regardless of the mountains of evidence I provided. All of what I spoke about always fell on deaf ears, as they seemed to not care about anything being said. In my opinion, if they cared then they would have listened and made the minimal changes requested for the short period of time that I visited.

Eventually, I learned that the convenience of their technology was more important than me visiting and therefore I stopped visiting.

The last time I visited, I kept my pain to myself and toughed it out for 3 hours. The symptoms I experienced were as follows:

1. Extreme brain fog
2. Twitching randomly
3. Vibrations throughout my entire body
4. Memory loss
5. Speech difficulty
6. A "melting" feeling
7. Shooting pain throughout my entire body
8. Numbness in my hands and feet
9. Tinnitus
10. An extreme migraine
11. Dizziness
12. Red eyes
13. Heart problems
14. Breathing difficulty
15. Extreme irritability and anger
16. Inflammation, especially in my brain/head
17. Overall feeling of sickness

Although the experience was a nightmare for me, I plastered a fake smile on my face and acted as if everything was fine. They had no clue and didn't ask how I was doing a single time. There were numerous moments during that visit that I thought I was going to pass out or die from the extreme EMF exposure but I pushed through the pain knowing that soon it would be over and I could leave. Being EHS with a family who refuses to understand is not why I told you that story. The reason why is because after leaving their house I immediately began detoxing.

Once at my low EMF home, the detoxing really set in, leading to the realization that a detox period occurs even after a single exposure. The first day I went through a period of extreme head pressure followed by massive migraines and uncontrollable body twitching. A draining sensation accompanied the symptoms, leaving me feeling as if I had just gone swimming and water was coming from my ears. The next few days I was more irritable than normal, and had flu like symptoms as well as minor swelling in my face. The total amount of time that the detox period occurred was 7 days and after that I stabilized back to my 90% health baseline.

After documenting my theory on detoxing from EMFs, I decided to put it to the test. I tested my theory by conducting a home inspection for someone who was EHS. Their home was nowhere near as bad as my parents, but then again nobody's home I have ever visited had been that bad. The symptoms I experienced while at that home inspection were as follows:

1. Brain fog
2. Difficulty breathing
3. Slight twitching
4. Brain inflammation

As you can see, the symptoms were minor in comparison to the ones experienced at my parents' home. After arriving home, my theory was confirmed as I experienced a detox period of approximately 2 days. During that time, I experienced the draining sensation, as well as a migraine and slight flu like symptoms.

My theory in regards to an EMF detox period was further confirmed upon experiencing similar symptoms after each home inspection conducted. Each and every time I visited a home with high levels of EMFs, there was a detox period lasting for approximately 2 days, depending on the severity of the exposure. After which, I always stabilized back to a 90% health baseline.

The reason why I believe there is an EMF detox period is because I have personally experienced and confirmed it. I believe that anyone who uses EMFs frequently will experience an original 14 day period of their body detoxing. That is however if they completely avoid EMFs for that 14 day period. After that, I believe the symptoms will go away, leaving the individual to establish a new baseline of health. For extreme cases, the detox period could last longer, but since I haven't met anyone with symptoms as severe as mine, I have nothing to base that theory on but my own experience. After that and while still avoiding EMFs, I believe the body then begins healing from the damage, which can take various amounts of time depending on the severity of the damage. For me it took approximately 9 months of prudent avoidance to reach the point of 90% health.

If by chance, exposure to EMFs occurs during the healing process, I believe minor detox periods will occur, lasting from 2-7 days. This however is all in regards to someone experiencing EHS, as I have not tested my theory on any other demographic. Shockingly, people who are not EHS are a lot less receptive to the idea of reducing their use of wireless technology. Even if I inform them that just because they can't feel it like I can, doesn't mean it's not doing the same thing.

Chapter 5

Other Things I've Tried

Throughout the entire process of regaining my health, there were numerous treatments that I tried. Some of them worked, while others did not. Below I have broken down the other things I've tried into sub sections in order to gain an idea of just how dedicated I was at getting better. Some of the treatments were for Lyme disease, some for mold illness, but most were centered around EHS.

In the beginning of the process of figuring out what exactly was wrong with me, I tried a multitude of various treatments and "things" in order to regain my health. This was all due to the fact that I was trying to figure out what was wrong with me on my own and without the help of anyone. It's not that I wouldn't have loved the help, it was because nobody believed that I was actually sick. Some of the things I tried, made me look crazy as you'll soon see, but I was desperate for answers and desperation may seem crazy to those who have never travelled that path.

Disulfiram

An over the counter pharmaceutical drug I was prescribed to take for Lyme disease was called "Disulfiram". A medication given to alcoholics that uses negative reinforcement to get them to quit drinking. Drinking alcohol while on this medication was said to cause instant vomiting. Therefore, anything that had alcohol in it (mouth wash, certain tinctures, etc.) was advised to avoid. Although its manufactured purpose was intended for alcoholics, it's off label use was said to help cure Lyme disease.

Disulfiram's claim to fame was that it was capable of killing the Lyme spirochete. However, this was a claim that was not well known within the medical community. I found this out first hand when I picked up my prescription at my local pharmacy. The pharmacist behind the counter was extremely judgmental when I asked to fill my prescription. Not that it was any of his business, but his first question for me was "oh, so you have a problem with alcohol?" My response was "no, I have Lyme disease." Not understanding that there was an off label use for the medication, he continued to insist that I had a problem with alcohol and that was the only thing that the medication was for. I insisted that it was not for its intended purpose and yet his response continued to remain the same. It was very frustrating.

After about 10 minutes of politely arguing with the pharmacist, he finally handed me my prescription. Not only was that confrontation embarrassing for me, but it put me in a really bad mood for the rest of the day. I really disliked the way he made me feel.

Leading me to research the medication on my own and see if there were other people with Lyme disease that had taken it. Clearly, I wasn't the only person taking disulfiram for Lyme disease, which became evident within minutes of research. Finding that out made me feel better.

That night, I took my first dose of the medication. Hours later, my body broke out into hives and became extremely swollen. My eyes were red and puffy, my lips felt as if they were going to explode, and my arms, chest and legs were covered in blotchy red spots. Not knowing what was happening to me, I contacted my girlfriend and informed her of my symptoms. She immediately stopped what she was doing, went to the store for Benadryl, and came over to take care of me. At the time, we had no idea that there was a correlation to the medication and assumed it was something that I ate.

After cancelling out the meals I ate that day and the possibility that it was an allergic reaction to food, we concluded that it was the medication. We then began looking through all of the additional medications I was taking to determine if there was any alcohol in them. The only medication we could find that contained alcohol was the "Yohimbe" that I was taking. However, I hadn't taken that medication in days, and the reaction that I experienced was unlike anything that others had experienced while taking disulfiram. Eventually the Benadryl kicked in, and the symptoms I was experiencing went away.

Being the stubborn guy that I am, I decided to take the medication again the next day. This time, I had zero reactions physically but felt more dizzy than normal. I then contacted my doctor at the Lyme and Cancer treatment center and asked if what I was experiencing was normal. His response was that it was a "herx reaction", which was normal and that my body was killing off the Lyme infection. For the next few days I continued to take the medication, experiencing light headedness and dizzy spells.

On the fifth day of taking the medication, my body broke out into hives once again. The thought of it being a herx reaction did not sit well with me due to the fact that it felt more like an allergic reaction. This time, my throat closed up and breathing became difficult, on top of the original symptoms. After taking Benadryl, the symptoms went away. I was then prescribed an "epi pen" after discussing my concerns of it being an allergic reaction with my doctor.

After the second time of breaking out into hives, I decided to not take the medication for a few days due to fear of possibly reacting to the medication. For five days, I was allergic reaction free and therefore concluded that it was related to the disulfiram. For some reason though, I decided to take the medication again on the sixth day and experienced the hives and throat closing once again. It wasn't bad enough to use the epi pen, and Benadryl seemed to reverse the symptoms. After that, I completely stopped taking disulfiram and have not taken again since.

To this day, I am still unsure as to why my body reacted the way that it did while taking disulfiram. I wasn't drinking alcohol, nor was I taking any medication that contained alcohol, and my diet remained the same. Maybe the doctor was correct about it being a herx reaction, or maybe I truly was allergic to the medication. One thing is for sure, I will not take that medication again.

Shower Filter

Think of a typical water filter that you would use to filter out the "bad stuff" from your tap drinking water. Now apply that same thought to the water coming out of your shower head. There are filters for your shower head that essentially do the same thing. In my opinion, if the water is not good enough for the inside of my body, why would I want to shower in it on the outside of my body? However, that's not the only reason why I switched to a filtered shower head. I switched because I randomly started getting sick while taking showers.

Each time I would shower, I would get light headed, my body would vibrate, and on occasion I would either pass out or throw up. In the past, showers had always left me feeling refreshed, then they became something I feared. I had no clue why all of a sudden, I was "allergic" to showering and after a few months of trying to push through my symptoms, I eventually stopped showering. By not showering I avoided the symptoms listed above.

Not showering though had its downsides, I started to stink. Not wanting to be the "stinky guy", I set out to try and figure out why the shower made me feel sick. I went through every EMF related test I could think of by testing the bathtubs electric field, magnetic field, radio frequencies in the bathroom and even my body voltage. All of which came back within the normal/safe range. After concluding it wasn't EMF related, I turned to the quality of the water for answers.

I purchased two separate water quality meters, one for testing the pH of the water, and one for testing the total dissolved solids (TDS). The results were through the roof on both meters, meaning that the water I was showering in was "less than sanitary". After that discovery, I researched possible ways to clean up my showers water and discovered that "dirty water" was extremely common. The solution I found was to use a shower filter.

Installing the shower filter was simple. All I had to do was twist off the old one and then twist the new one on, taking only 2 minutes. Once it was installed, I then retested the water quality with my pH meter and TDS meter, which showed that the water was now safe. After that, showering no longer caused any negative symptoms and once again became a safe place for me.

From what I learned while researching, I may have been suffering from multiple chemical sensitivity (MCS). Apparently, people with EHS are more often than not also chemically sensitive. By replacing my shower head for a filtered one, my problem was solved.

Detox Baths

Taking baths was never all that amusing for me, I preferred showers. Discovering detox baths changed my perspective and quickly became one of my favorite treatments. I'm not exactly sure where I read about the exact mixture of ingredients I used, but somehow, I figured it out and have perfected it over the years. The ingredients used in my detox baths were as follows:

1. 2lb bag of pink Himalayan Epsom salts
2. 2.5lb Baking soda
3. 32fl.oz Hydrogen peroxide
4. A few drops of tea tree oil
5. 1 cap full of lavender bubble bath (depending on time of day, for relaxation purposes)

The 2lb bag of pink Himalayan Epsom salts was used for its rich quantity of magnesium. Without going into too much detail, EMFs deplete the body of magnesium, therefore by bathing in it, it soaks into the skin from the outside. On days where I have a high exposure of EMFs, I double up the amount of Epsom salts to a total of 4lbs.

As far as the other ingredients go, they act together to pull the toxins out of the body. With EHS, my detoxification pathways are faulty, and by aiding the body in the form of a bath, detoxification can occur. For approximately 6 months, I took a 1 hour detox bath every single day. They helped relieve my body of physical pain, the random twitching stopped, and my brain fog decreased. After that, my body's ability to detox improved, which led to less baths needed.

Today, I am on an "as needed" basis regarding my detox baths. If I have a high exposure to EMFs, part of my routine for recovery includes a detox bath. Other than that, if I feel that a detox bath is needed, I take one. On average I now take approximately 3 detox baths per week.

Shielded Clothing

When I first realized that I was EHS, the shielded clothing market was minimal. On top of that, the market that did exist contained options that were far from fashionable. This meant that I had to wear the options available, or purchase faraday fabric and make my own articles of clothing. I did both. Years later, the EMF protection clothing market exploded. Purchasing any article of clothing with EMF protection is now just a click away.

I have tried a large majority of the EMF protection clothing options available over the years and have determined that some work, but most do not. The intended purpose of shielded clothing is to shield your body from the harmful radio frequencies present in our world today. Shielded clothing does not protect your body from Electric Fields, Magnetic Fields, or dirty electricity. In order to understand how the shielded clothing works, I developed a rather simple explanation.

Radio Frequencies are basically waves of energy traveling through the air. These waves are relatively small, but are powerful enough to penetrate through various types of materials. By using conductive materials that are tightly woven together, creating a net almost, the radio frequencies are unable to penetrate through and are displaced over the large conductive area. This in turn, prevents the radio frequencies from penetrating the body. This material is effective enough that if you were to wrap your cell phone up tightly within it, it would not receive a signal.

The fabric is also used in astronaut suits to protect them from the harmful radiation present in space.

However, like I stated earlier, not all of the options available work. Some have been poorly designed and result in turning the material into more of an antenna, attracting radio frequencies and not protecting the body as claimed. Below I have listed the main areas I looked for before purchasing any article of clothing:

1. **Shielding percentage:** This can be one of the more confusing and tricky areas regarding shielded material. The material may be 99% effective at shielding radio frequencies, but the frequency at which it blocks is low. Let's say it blocks 99% at 100mhz, which from an uninformed perspective seems pretty good. However, radio frequencies today exceed 8ghz, which is a lot higher of a frequency than 100mhz. For the material to be most effective, you want the shielding percentage to be as high as possible, as well as tested against the highest frequencies.
2. **Attenuation:** This refers to the surface conductivity of the material and is typically referred to in "Decibel level (dB)" or "Ohms". The higher the dB or Ohms, the higher the

conductivity. The higher the conductivity, the more beneficial the material is at dispensing radio frequencies.
3. **Lab tested:** If the product has been tested inside of a lab for its effectiveness, then it will state that it has been lab tested. I always looked up the labs to verify if they actually existed, and half the time they didn't. Which meant I wasn't going to purchase the product.

Wearing shielded clothing has been extremely beneficial for me during the healing process. In fact, shielded clothing has been so beneficial, that I continue to wear it to this day. As much as I'd like to say that wearing shielded clothing is 100% effective at protecting the body from harmful radio frequencies, that simply wouldn't be the truth. In my opinion, the truth is that it is only protects to a certain level. The high amounts of radio frequencies in today's world are far too high to expect complete protection. Therefore, complete protection is not something that should be expected. For me, shielded clothing protects my body from about 40-50% of radio frequencies, even if the material I'm wearing states its protection levels are above 99%.

The symptoms in which I have noticed a significant improvement in since wearing shielded clothing are as follows:

1. Reduction in headaches and migraines
2. Improvement in memory
3. Less numbness and tingling in body
4. Less brain fog
5. Reduction in speech problems

6. Less body weakness
7. Improvement in energy
8. Reduction in anger issues and irritability
9. Less vibrations in body
10. Reduction in sore joints
11. Reduction in tinnitus
12. Easier to focus and concentrate
13. Less anxiety and nervousness
14. Lower blood pressure
15. Reduction in feeling of light headedness
16. Reduction in heart problems (irregular heartbeats, feeling as if having heart attack)
17. More feeling in parts of body that had unknowingly to me been numb
18. Easier to fall asleep and stay asleep
19. Ability to dream as well as remember what I dreamt about
20. Improvement in overall well-being

For those of you who are wondering what I wear for shielded clothing in order to achieve the above results, I have created a list below. Although the listed articles of shielded clothing are what I wear every single day, I cannot recommend any of them. The list is for informative purposes only and should not be seen as me recommending them. I am not your doctor and cannot make any recommendations, otherwise I'd get in trouble. So, do whatever you please with the information I am sharing below.

1. **Shielded hat.** For this I took my favorite hat and taped the entire inside with faraday tape. The tape I used was called "TitanRF tape". There are other options for hats that are already made with shielding capabilities, but

they stand out too much for me. Instead, I prefer for people to not know I am wearing EMF protection and chose to make my own using shielded tape. I wear this hat every second of the day, unless I'm showering or sleeping.
2. **Shielded beanie.** I wear a shielded protection beanie while I sleep, every single night. The one I use is from a company called "Lvfeier". They are silver in color and can be sewn under a normal beanie in order to look more fashionable.
3. **Shielded tank top.** The tank top I use was one of the first shielded articles of clothing that I purchased. It is from a company called "OURSURE", and is gold in color. I wear this during the day, and at night while I sleep.
4. **Shielded t-shirt.** On top of my shielded tank top, I also wear a shielded t-shirt from a company called "Lambs". The only thing I don't like about this t-shirt is that the neck area doesn't bounce back after washing it, resulting in a really loose fitting neck line. It is black on the outside and gold on the inside, making it a very inconspicuous option for shielded clothing. Due to the neck being so loose, I choose to wear a regular shirt on top of that, using it more like an undershirt. I wear this during the day, and at night while I sleep.
5. **Shielded underwear.** I wear shielded underwear from a company called "Lambs". I have tried every single other pair of shielded underwear that was available at the time of writing this, and found that these are by far my favorite and protect my body the best.

They are black on the outside and gold on the inside. I wear these during the day, and at night while I sleep.

6. **Shielded tights.** The tights I wear are for woman, because they don't make any for men. They are from a company called "YShield". They are gold in color, and are thin enough to fit underneath a regular pair of pants. I wear them during the day, and at night while I sleep.

7. **Shielded socks.** The socks I wear are from a company called "LessEMF". They are gray in color and are only offered in sizes 8-10. I wear a size 13 shoe, so they are a little small on me, but they still go above my ankle. The only thing I don't like about these socks is that there is a little metal button clip on each of them. The clip is for a grounding cable to be attached to them. I do not use the metal button clip and dislike that it is there. There was another pair of shielded socks that I wore for a very long time from a company called "Silverell", but I have not been able to find them since purchasing my original three pairs. I believe they have been discontinued. They were black in color, but were dress socks and were uncomfortable to wear with regular shoes. The soles ended up wearing out completely, resulting in a loss of shielding effectiveness. I prefer my gray pair though, so I'm not complaining. I wear my gray pair of shielded socks during the day, and at night while I sleep.

8. **Shielded insoles.** These are not available anywhere online or in stores, because they

don't exist. I made them myself and use them in any pair of shoes that I'm wearing for the day. What I did was purchase comfortable insoles, as well as "TitanRF tape", and taped the entire bottom of the insole. Then all I did was slip the insole into my shoe, and I was protected from the bottom up.

9. **Blue light blocking glasses.** The market for blue light blocking glasses is large. The ones I originally purchased were from a company called "Anrri". They are black in color, and plastic framed. However, I then purchased 60 pairs from China from a company that no longer exists. These blue light blocking glasses are the absolute best I have owned and put my original ones to shame. I wear them all day, especially while driving. They do not block radio frequencies, only blue light from screens like cell phones, televisions, and computers.

10. **Shielded glasses.** These are different from my blue light blocking glasses, as they are not actual glasses and don't contain any actual glass. They are from a company called "LessEMF". Rather than glass, there is a conducive metal mesh wiring. They are black in color and look pretty funny on my face. I use these anytime I feel as if my eyes may be exposed to radio frequencies. I either wear these or my blue light blocking glasses while driving.

11. **Shielded scarf.** This was something else that I made due to the fact that there wasn't anything out on the market at the time. The fabric purchased was from a company called "LessEMF", but this specific fabric is no longer

available. It is gold in color, and is see through. I wrap the scarf around my neck while driving, during the day, and at night while I sleep.

12. **Shielded blanket.** This blanket is my absolute favorite product that I own. In fact, I own three of them. One for underneath me while I sleep, one for the top of me, and one for my significant other. It is about the size of a twin sized comforter, beige on the top side and gold on the bottom. It's from a company called "Summit Bioceuticals". I sleep with this blanket every single night, wrap myself up in it if the radio frequencies are high during the day, and even bring it with me wherever I travel.

13. **Shielded fitted sheet and top sheet.** Prior to purchasing the blanket listed above, these sheets were my favorite. They are white in color and look like normal sheets, which was nice. They are from a company called "LessEMF". I sleep with these sheets every single night. The only bad thing about these sheets is that if you wash them too often, they lose shielding effectiveness. So, I put an additional sheet on top of the fitted sheet in order to avoid having to wash it as often. By doing this, the shielding effectiveness has stayed intact.

14. **Shielded Pillowcase.** This pillowcase is one of my favorite products, especially because it's easy to travel with. It's from a company called "LessEMF" and is white in color. I first put it on my pillow, then put an additional pillowcase on top of that in order to protect it

from having to be washed as frequently. I sleep with this pillowcase every single night.
15. **Shielded seat cushion.** Taking the same fabric that I used to make my shielded scarf (LessEMF), I also made my own shielded seat cushion for my car. I purchased one of the memory foam type seat cushions that has a cover that zips off, as well as the shielded fabric. Then I unzipped the seat cushion, took out the memory foam, wrapped it in the shielded fabric, and then put it back inside. From the outside, it looks like a normal black seat cushion, but on the inside, it is wrapped in gold colored shielded fabric. I use this every single time I drive, as well as if I'm ever in a vehicle that is not my own.
16. **Shielded key fob holder.** This product was from a company called "TitanRF". It is a little pouch lined with faraday fabric, that I put my car keys into, when not in use. On the outside it's black, and on the inside it's gold in color. While my key fob is inside the holder, my car does not read it and my car will not start.

As far as protection for my cell phone goes, I firmly believe they are a waste of money. I have tried various pouches, which have all worked to some extent but I prefer to just put my phone on airplane mode. It's free, and it doesn't require any additional product. My cell phone remains on airplane mode 99% of the time and therefore a pouch is not needed.

At one point I also had a shielded bed canopy that looked like a mosquito net. It was purchased from LessEMF, and was white in color. I stopped using it because touching it made me feel sick and touching it was inevitable. Also, I did have a shielded sleeping bag that I used a lot, but once I purchased the blanket, it proved to be useless. Compared to the blanket, the sleeping bag did very little for me. I purchased the sleeping bag from a company called "LeBlock" and it was gray in color.

Although the list above is extensive, I do wear all of the products every single day. None of them require grounding, and are easily hidden under my normal clothes. Without shielded clothing, I begin feeling my symptoms coming back within minutes of a high exposure of radio frequencies.

Smart Meter Cover

Smart meters are a device located on your home that reads how much electricity you use. Your usage is then sent from your smart meter to your utility company through a wireless radio frequency transmission. Before smart meters you had an analog meter that a utility worker would have to manually check each month. While this new technology definitely saved utility companies money by not having to pay workers to manually check your usage, it also created a whole new problem. Unlike the old analog meters, new smart meters send your usage through pulsed radio frequency waves at levels well above what is considered safe. The pulsed radio frequency waves emitted by smart meters occur hundreds if not thousands of times per day and are capable of penetrating the walls of your home.

Using my radio frequency meter, I was able to

determine the strength of each pulse as well as the rate at which the pulses occur. Not only was I able to track the pulses from the smart meter on my home, but also the pulses coming from each and every one of neighbors' homes. This was accomplished by standing inside of my garage or backyard while pointing my radio frequency meter at any visible smart meter.

While tracking the pulses coming from the smart meters on my home as well as my neighbors' homes, I noticed a pattern and developed three separate categories based on the results:

1. Daytime usage: 7:00AM-6:00PM
2. Nighttime usage: 6:00PM-7:00AM
3. Weekend usage: Friday 6:00PM- Monday 7:00AM

During the day while my neighbors were at work, their smart meters pulsed an average of once every 27 seconds, spiking over 2,000 µW/m2 on my radio frequency meter. However, each homes smart meter pulse occurred at different times and were not on the same schedule. This resulted in an overlap of pulses where at least one homes smart meter was pulsing every second of the day. My assumption was that even though they were not home, their devices were still plugged in using electricity and therefore usage was being tracked via their smart meters. With everything unplugged inside my home (except my refrigerator), and a majority of my power cut off at the breaker box, my smart meter pulsed an average of once every 3 minutes. All of the smart meters in my neighborhood were the same, and two of my immediate neighbors had 2 smart meters due to their solar panels. Comparing my home to my neighbors' homes was how I was able to reach the conclusion that it was electricity usage related.

At around 6:00PM when my neighbors get home from work, their electricity usage increases, resulting in an increase of pulsed radio frequencies coming from their smart meters. My assumption here was that whenever you use something inside your home that requires electricity, the smart meter tracks it and sends it to your utility company immediately. At night these pulses occurred on average once every 3 seconds from my neighbors' homes. Just like during the day, the pulses overlapped at night with at least one of my neighbors' smart meters pulsing every second. Stepping out of my garage and into my courtyard at night, the constant background levels of pulsed radio frequencies coming from smart meters is 1,000 µW/m2, spiking to well over 2,000 µW/m2 every second. My homes smart meter remained pulsing an average of once every 3 minutes (2,000 µW/m2), with an occasional less intense pulse in between (500 µW/m2).

During the weekend all of my neighbors were home, resulting in more electricity use and more pulsed radio frequency waves coming from their smart meters. These pulses occurred once every 3 seconds during the day and night during the entire weekend. Since my electricity usage remained about the same regardless of the day of week, my smart meter continued to pulse once every 3 minutes, even on the weekend.

For comparison purposes, my iPhone 8 puts off 5 µW/m2 when it is on but not "lit up". When I tap the screen or "wake it up", it pulses to around 1,000 µW/m2. When I receive a text message, it pulses to around 1,500 µW/m2. When I receive a phone call, it pulses to over 2,000 µW/m2.

The symptoms I experienced from the high levels of radio frequency pulses coming from my smart meter as well as my neighbors' smart meters were primarily related to my heart, brain and breathing. My heart would beat erratically and irregular whenever a pulse would occur. I would immediately get brain fog, lose my train of thought, forget simple words while speaking, suffer from short term memory loss, and feel my brain swell. My breathing would become labored and sometimes it would even become difficult to catch my breath. The explanation I would always give would be that I felt as if I were hiking an extremely high mountain, or submerged deeply inside a pool. That was all until I purchased a smart meter guard.

The smart meter guard was basically a cover made out of tightly woven, conductive metal fabric, that slips over your smart meter creating somewhat of a faraday cage. Since my smart meter was located on the outside of my garage, I also placed a large piece of faraday fabric on the opposite side of it. This piece of faraday fabric was for extra protection and was located on the inside of my garage, right behind where the smart meter was located. The smart meter guard doesn't eliminate the radio frequencies but rather, reduces them. Completely enclosing the smart meter with faraday fabric would result in zero signal getting out and the utility company knocking on the front door. With the smart meter guard the signal still gets out, but instead of radio frequencies exceeding 2,000 µW/m2, my highest reading went down to 200 µW/m2.

The symptoms related to smart meter exposure went away after installing the smart meter guard and faraday fabric on the inside of my garage. Unfortunately, that's only the case on the inside of my house in the room furthest away from my smart meter. Outside of my home, my neighbors' smart meters still pulse every 3 to 27 seconds depending on the day, and my heart, brain and breathing related symptoms come back within minutes of stepping outside. At least I now know the correlation between those specific symptoms and smart meter radio frequency exposure.

For those of you wondering why I didn't try and contact my utility company to "opt out" of the smart meter on my home, I tried and was told "my neighborhood doesn't offer that service." Ridiculous, I know. I also thought of discussing with my neighbors the dangers associated with their smart meters and offering to purchase smart meter guards for their homes, but I live in a rather "rough" neighborhood and have been too scared of being called crazy. Maybe one day I'll get over my fears associated with the stigma EHS carries and freely discuss the dangers of EMFs with everyone I can. Until that day comes, I'll just keep writing and doing whatever I can to protect myself from my neighbors' smart meters.

Since writing this section, there are now smart meters for water, gas, and electricity. All monitoring usage through pulsed radio frequencies.

Driving

One area that I have had a very difficult time tackling is protection from EMFs while driving. Cars today are equipped with Wi-Fi and Bluetooth, which means escaping radio frequencies is nearly impossible. Each car that I pass while driving is connected to their Bluetooth devices, and some are even connected to Wi-Fi. Making the radio frequency readings coming off their cars just as high as the cell towers I pass.

Cell towers are everywhere in today's world. By doing a search on "antennasearch.com", you'd be shocked at just how many there are surrounding your home, office, and even your children's schools. All of which, I pass while driving, getting exposure levels well above safe limits.

The car that I drive is a 2016 Jeep Grand Cherokee. I have disabled the Bluetooth option, and do not have Wi-Fi. Here is a list of things that I have done to my car in order to shield myself from EMFs:

1. **Tinted windows:** I tinted every single window in my car, even the front windshield. This has helped shield some of the radio frequencies coming through my windows from outside sources. To be honest, it only blocks about 5% of EMFs, but that's better than nothing in my opinion.
2. **Shielded seat cushion:** I purchased one of the

memory foam type seat cushions that has a cover that zips off, as well as the shielded fabric. Then I unzipped the seat cushion, took out the memory foam, wrapped it in the shielded fabric, and then put it back inside. From the outside, it looks like a normal black seat cushion, but on the inside it is wrapped in gold colored shielded fabric. This has helped somewhat while driving, but not enough to make a significant difference.

3. **Tint on display screen:** The screen that my car came with was extremely bright and during my sensitivity to light phase, it was too much for me to handle. Therefore, I purchased a sheet of tint, and applied it over the screen. It helped tremendously with my light sensitivity while driving my car at night.

4. **Tinfoil under floormats:** Prior to understanding the difference between radio frequencies and magnetic fields, I placed tinfoil under my floormats because I thought it would prevent the magnetic fields from entering through my feet. Although tinfoil only blocks radio frequencies, I chose to leave it under my floormats because you can't see them, and for some reason they make me feel better. For this, all I did was purchase tinfoil tape, flipped my floormats over, taped the entire bottom of them, flipped them back over, and that was it. From the top, you cannot see the tinfoil at all.

That's it. That's all I've done. There aren't many options on protecting yourself from EMFs while driving. I have thought about the correlation between my surges in anger and the number of EMFs I'm around while driving and believe shielded vehicles would be beneficial at lowering road rage. That however, is just my opinion.

While driving inside my car, I also do not use my phone at all. It remains on airplane mode, even while using my GPS. This was taught to me by my girlfriend, and is actually very easy to do. Below are the steps I take to use GPS if needed, while on airplane mode:

1. While the phone is on and not on airplane mode, load the location you are going to in the GPS.
2. Once it has loaded, press start/go and wait for it to begin.
3. Then turn your phone on airplane mode and you're set.

The only downside to using your phones GPS while on airplane mode, is that if you make a wrong turn it doesn't always reload an alternate route. When that happens, I pull over and turn my phone off of airplane mode and let the route calculate an alternative route. Then I place my phone back on airplane mode and continue driving. This is a much safer way to travel for me.

As far as other thoughts I've had regarding my car goes, I've had many. Here is a list of things that I have thought could potentially work at protecting myself while driving:

1. **Shielded window tint:** On the website

LessEMF, they sell radio frequency blocking window tint. My only concern would be that if I used that tint, the only area of my car that would be shielded would be my windows. If radio frequencies made their way into my car, they would then bounce around, unable to escape from the inside of my windows and ultimately raising my exposure.
2. **Shielded fabric:** I thought about purchasing shielded fabric and going to an interior car upholstery company. They would then upholster the entire inside of my car with shielded fabric. This would be very expensive, and most of the options for fabric come in gold or silver, which would be too obvious for my preference.
3. **Shielded paint:** The company YShield makes paint for your home that shields from radio frequencies. My thought was to paint the inside of my car with this paint. That was until I learned that the paint must be grounded in order to work to its full potential. Since grounding my car is impossible to do while driving, and home paint isn't the same as car paint, I gave up on that thought.
4. **Nonmagnetic tires:** Apparently, tires today have a metal mesh inside of them that when you drive, creates a magnetic field. This field was tested on my NFA1000 meter and gave off extremely high magnetic field readings that extended all the way up into my driver and passenger seats. I didn't test my rear tires because I assumed they were the same as my front ones. I would like to purchase tires without metal mesh inside of them in order to

prevent exposing myself to high Magnetic Fields.
5. **Full body suit:** On the website LessEMF, there is a full body shielded suit that looks sort of like a contamination coverall suit. It is white in color and offers very high shielding from radio frequencies. The only reason why I haven't worn this while driving (or purchased it) is because I don't want to look crazy. However, with people wearing face masks everywhere they go due to COVID-19, it may not look as crazy as I was thinking.

As you can see, I've thought of a lot of options to shield myself from EMFs while driving, none of which are easily accomplished. Unfortunately, this has prevented me from driving as much as I would like to and even prevented me from getting in other people's cars. Hopefully one day there will be an easier way to stay protected from harmful EMF radiation while driving.

Dirty Electricity Filters

While researching EMFs I came across the concept of dirty electricity. So, I purchased a dirty electricity meter to determine if my home had any. To my surprise, the dirty electricity levels in my home were 10 times higher than the recommended safe level. At the time I had no clue as to just how bad dirty electricity is to be around, let alone while trying to heal my body.

Dirty electricity is created by excess oscillation and spikes of frequencies exceeding 60hz while traveling from one point to another. In basic terms, it means that rather than having a steady stream of 60hz electricity flowing through your walls, you receive spikes of higher levels of electricity than is needed to power your devices. This in turn can cause your devices to malfunction or even worse, cause adverse health effects in your body.

In my home, the meter I used to determine my levels of dirty electricity used millivolts as the unit of measurement. As long as the electricity coming through my walls was under 25 millivolts (mV), you were okay. Using the device was easy. All you had to do was plug it into the wall, and it shows you exactly how much dirty electricity is coming through your wiring. It also had an audible function that let you hear what the electricity sounds like. Most of the time it sounded like static, but on a few occasions, I could literally hear what my neighbors were watching on their televisions. This was due to the fact that their devices created dirty electricity, which then traveled from their home and into mine.

The first time I plugged the meter into an outlet in my home, it read 250mV. However, that was just one outlet checked. I spent a full hour checking each and every outlet inside my home, documenting my results. The worst outlet was closest to my kitchen, which was putting off 350mV. The lowest reading was located in the area furthest from my kitchen, 245mV. Upstairs at the top of my staircase, the reading was 260mV but the sound was different. The sound coming from the meter was a preacher talking about Jesus. I could hear word for word what this preacher was saying, it was very eye opening. I knew at that point that I had a problem with dirty electricity and began researching ways to mitigate it.

As far as what could be done to the inside of my home to lower my dirty electricity levels, there wasn't a whole lot that could be done without hiring a professional. Therefore, I opted for the cheapest option that could be accomplished on my own and ordered "dirty electricity filters". The filters I ordered were from a company called GreenWave. They arrived at my front door in less than a week and were extremely easy to install. All I had to do was plug them into the wall outlet and that was it. However, one was not enough to clean up the amount of dirty electricity I had, so I had to purchase 16 in total.

The dirty electricity filters work by cleaning up the electricity coming through your wiring while creating a more constant and steadier stream of clean electricity. I'm not exactly sure how these devices work, but from personal experience and measurement, they work.

The best part about having the meter as well as the filter, is that you can visibly see the difference the filters make. Here are the steps I took to lower my dirty electricity with the filters:

1. Plug in dirty electricity meter to the top plug in your outlet.
2. See the reading on the top line of the meter. Mine was 350mV.
3. Plug in the dirty electricity filter in the bottom plug of the outlet while the meter is still plugged into the top.

4. See the reading on the bottom line of the meter. Mine dropped to 20mV.
5. The meter then shows an additional line showing the total reduction. Mine was a 99% reduction.

It was that easy and took less than 20 minutes to install all 16 filters inside my home. Most of the readings in my home after that were a 98% reduction or more, from what they were prior to installing the dirty electricity filters. The night I installed the filters, I was actually able to fall asleep. That in turn, started my new obsession with eliminating as much dirty electricity as possible within my home. The other steps I took to eliminate dirty electricity were:

1. Get rid of all fluorescent light bulbs. These apparently create large amounts of dirty electricity by turning on and off thousands of times per second.
2. Unplug everything in my home that I wasn't using. This prevents any new dirty electricity being created by the devices that are plugged in.
3. Avoid using any ungrounded plugs. Grounded plugs have three prongs, ungrounded have only two. These create massive amounts of dirty electricity because they are ungrounded. The excess electricity then floats through the air invisibly and is attracted to your body. That raises your body voltage, which should be zero.

Everything that I did to lower the dirty electricity within my home was only one piece of the EMF puzzle. The fact that I was extremely sick still made it difficult to see major improvements in my health but the small things I did notice were documented. Below is a list of the improvements I did notice after lowering my dirty electricity:

1. Less dizziness
2. Easier to fall asleep
3. Less brain fog
4. Less headaches
5. Less vibrating feeling in my body
6. More energy
7. Waking up easier

To this day, I still use dirty electricity filters inside my home as well as anytime I have attempted to stay at a hotel.

Floating

Floating is essentially the same thing as sitting in a bathtub full of Epsom salts. The main difference between your bathtub at home and a facility for "floating" is the quantity of Epsom salts. The facility I went to used approximately 5,000 pounds of Epsom salts.

The facility itself was small, and contained 10 individual treatment rooms. Seven of the rooms were "floating" rooms, two were neurotherapy rooms, and one room was a sauna. After checking in at the front desk, you are walked back to one of the floating rooms, told to take your shoes off prior to entering, and then you step inside the room.

Stepping inside the room, the first thing you see is a large white pod situated near the back wall. It was approximately 10 feet long, 5 feet wide, 5 feet tall, and looked sort of like a device out of an alien movie. It was equipped with glowing blue lights, and opened up in the center revealing glowing blue water inside. The rest of the room was completely covered in bathroom tile from floor to ceiling, and had a small shower area opposite the pod.

After getting undressed, you are instructed to put noise cancelling ear plugs inside your ears, shower without soap, and then step inside the pod. Once inside the pod, you close the top and are completely enclosed inside. From the inside it looks like a bathtub with a roof on top of it. Since there was 5,000 pounds of Epsom salts inside the water, you float. After approximately 1 minute, the blue lights turn off and you are left inside the pod feeling weightless, with no sound, and in complete darkness. It is total sensory deprivation.

The total floating treatment lasts around 45 minutes. Once completed, the blue lights slowly turn back on, and the pod hatch slowly opens. Then you get out of the pod, take a shower with soap this time (in order to wash off all the Epsom salts) and get dressed.

The experience of being inside the pod was magical for me. I felt amazing floating weightlessly and usually fell asleep within minutes of the lights turning off. My only complaint was having to step out of the pod and onto the tile flooring. Being EHS, I could feel my symptoms begin to flare the moment my feet hit the ground. Then having to stand under the vast amount of fluorescent lights made me feel dizzy and extremely disoriented. Sometimes it would take me 30 minutes just to get dressed due to the brain fog. Although it was not an ideal location for someone with EHS, the benefits of soaking in the magnesium rich Epsom salts were worth it for me. I continued to go to the floating facility for an additional 14 times, attempting to heal my body with the 5,000 pounds of Epsom salts.

If the facility itself switched the fluorescent lights out for incandescent bulbs, and lowered the number of EMFs, I would highly recommend floating. Filling your bathtub at home with 5,000 pounds of Epsom salts is far too expensive.

Chiropractor

Going to the chiropractor was not my idea, but I'm a team player, so I went. The office was located downtown, in a sort of "strip mall" of offices. Getting there was easy, but walking inside was like stepping into a nightmare. There were EMF devices everywhere. At the front door there was a large flat screen tv that was on and connected to Wi-Fi. There was an iPad at the front desk that was used to check me in. The table where you lay to get adjusted had another iPad connected to Wi-Fi, the chiropractors iPhone, and a Bluetooth wireless speaker, all within inches of where I was supposed to lay my head.

It was horrible, but I kept my mouth shut and dealt with the pain. I went there a total of three times, without explaining that I was EHS (out of fear of embarrassment). On the third time, I couldn't take it anymore and decided to share my illness with the chiropractor.

The first approach I took was by telling him "I'm electrically hypersensitive, which means I'm essentially allergic to electricity." That approach was clearly wrong and I instantly regretted it as he stared at me like I was crazy. Then I tried another approach where I actually explained what EHS was. His response was to not respond at all and once again, stared at me like I was crazy. Then I tried going the science route, which he finally responded "maybe it's a frequency thing" and began to ask me if I had ever gone to someone to try and "fix my reaction to the frequency." Clearly, I wasn't explaining things right because his response was said in a mocking voice with an undertone of sarcasm. That was the last time I went there.

To make things clear, I didn't stop going because I wasn't seeing results, because I was. I stopped going because of the way the chiropractor treated me. How simple would it have been for the chiropractor to turn off his Wi-Fi and other EMF emitting devices while I was there? I know I was only one customer, with a condition unfamiliar to most, but just because you don't understand something, doesn't make it not real. If I reacted negatively to cigarette smoke, and the office was filled with people smoking, only two options are possible in my opinion: 1- stop smoking while I'm there, or 2- don't stop smoking and lose a customer. He unfortunately, lost a customer.

Parasites

One night while lying in bed with my girlfriend, a shooting pain entered my stomach and left me feeling as if it were going to explode. My stomach expanded and contracted, until I eventually ended up in the bathroom. I thought it was food poisoning or possibly a stomach bug, but I was wrong. Half way through using the bathroom, I felt a "worm-like" feeling wiggling out of my butt. Not knowing what to do and freaking out at the same time, I grabbed a piece of toilet paper, reached behind me and pulled out what was wiggling. Immediately I swung open the bathroom door and shouted to my girlfriend "I think I just passed a parasite!" After that, I snapped a picture for proof, and then flushed it down the toilet.

Lying in bed after that, my stomach pain had disappeared but the thought of what had happened left me feeling concerned. Randomly, my girlfriend and I began talking about colon hydrotherapy and how some machines have UV lights to show when a parasite passes. In that moment, everything clicked.

In the past I had used a black light on my stool for reasons I don't recall, and remember seeing streaks of blue and red glowing like strands of spaghetti. Telling my girlfriend this, left her shouting "why didn't you tell me this before?!" Apparently, some parasites glow under UV light and your stool, if parasite free, shouldn't glow.

The next day I began a parasite cleanse and began carrying a UV light with me each time I used the bathroom. The parasite cleanse consisted of taking a bunch of pills, and upping the amount of colon hydrotherapies to two a week. About an hour after taking the pills, I would feel the effects start to kick in. My stomach would always feel upset, and then 15 minutes later I would have to use the restroom. It was like clockwork.

A few days later I passed a 6" parasite that glowed blue and was even still moving in the toilet after exiting my body. With each day that passed, I felt the parasite cleanse working more and more.

VGCCs

While reading and researching EMFs, I stumbled across a pattern in the text. Each and every article or book stated that EMFs affect the Voltage Gated Calcium Channels (VGCC). This causes excess calcium to flood the body, which causes adverse effects. Some of the books even suggested taking calcium channel blockers in order to temporarily fix the issue. So, I obtained a prescription for a low dose calcium channel blocker and decided to experiment on myself.

If something as simple as a single pill would place a band aid on my symptoms, I was willing to try it. From the moment I picked up the prescription, to the second I got home, I was anxious. I was anxious because the research was compelling and I was ready to find a cure.

Prior to taking the first dose, I tracked my blood pressure, SpO2, and heart rate. They were all within normal range. Then I took the first pill and sat down with a pen and paper waiting for anything to happen. Honestly, I thought all my symptoms were going to disappear but that's not exactly what happened.

After approximately 30 minutes of sitting and waiting, I began to feel strange. My heart was beating different, my body became flushed with redness, and my breathing was slow and shallow. My blood pressure dropped, my SpO2 dropped and my heart rate increased. I regretted taking the pill in that moment and should have known that there wasn't a quick fix.

The symptoms related to taking the pill lasted for another few hours. After that I knew even more that if I were going to heal my body, it wouldn't be from temporary band aids like calcium channel blockers.

Dry Brushing

Throughout being sick, a strange "draining" sensation would occur in various parts of my body. Sometimes it happened in my ears, but mainly happened in my arms, spine (especially near my C7), and in the back of my head. The draining happened at random times, and until I figured out it was related to my lymphatic fluid, I described the feeling as "warm sand slowly dripping down the inside of my skin."

The discovery of dry brushing was a game changer. By brushing the skin around where the draining feeling typically occurred, I would begin to feel a "pins and needles" sensation, followed by the draining. From my understanding, EMFs caused my detoxification pathways to become clogged, which meant my lymphatic system wasn't working properly. By dry brushing, I was able to help my body circulate the lymphatic fluid and ultimately prevent buildups or clogging from occurring.

After a few months of dry brushing daily, the draining feeling disappeared and only occurs after a major EMF exposure. Even then, if I dry brush immediately after, it goes away fairly quick. Dry brushing is now a part of my daily routine. For prevention purposes and because it feels good.

Mold Candles

Being that my life revolved around finding a cure for what was wrong with me, I stumbled across candles that claimed to eliminate mold spores from the air.

Since I had abnormally high mold levels in my body at the time, I figured they would help prevent additional exposures. I was right.

Upon lighting them for the first time, they made the air in my house "fresher" and soon became somewhat of an obsession. I continued to order them over and over for two simple reasons:

1. They didn't last that long (8 hours or so)
2. They worked well

After a few months of using the candles daily, my girlfriend had the idea to make our own. That's when I began researching essential oils that eliminate mold spores. The three top essential oils found were: clove, thyme, and cinnamon.

Using essential oils in candles isn't effective though, so I opted for "fragrance oils" instead. After receiving all three, my girlfriend began making our very own mold candles. The process itself was simple.

- **Step 1:** Find a glass container that you want to use for the candle. We used "Oui Yogurt" glass containers because they were the perfect size.
- **Step 2:** Buy the wick and make sure it's the one with the metal piece on the bottom as well as the one with the sticky piece on the bottom of the metal. This is so that it actually sticks to the bottom of the glass.
- **Step 3:** Buy soy wax or beeswax. The other types of wax are cheaper but they are too toxic and bad to inhale.
- **Step 4:** Buy clove, thyme, and cinnamon "fragrance oil". You can choose to buy just one of the fragrance oils if you would like, but I prefer to use all three. Make sure not to purchase "essential oils" because they are not meant for candle making and dissolve extremely fast.
- **Step 5:** Get a metal pot that you don't care about ruining. We use a separate glass container rather than a pot. Make sure not to use the same container the candle will end up in, for melting the wax.
- **Step 6:** Place the soy wax or beeswax inside of the metal pot or glass container. They usually come in pellet form.
- **Step 7:** Turn the oven on to 200 degrees

Fahrenheit.

- **Step 8:** Place the metal pot or glass container with the wax inside it, on a baking sheet and put it inside the oven.
- **Step 9:** After about 20/30 minutes, check on the wax to see if it has melted. If it has, put on oven mitts and take it out from the oven.
- **Step 10:** Place the wick in the glass container you chose for your candle, making sure it's secure on the bottom of the container.
- **Step 11:** Pour the wax into the glass container, with the wick secured to the bottom. In order to keep the wick from moving while you pour in the wax, make sure you use some sort of wick stabilizer. We used a store-bought stabilizer that holds the wick in the center by resting on top of the container.
- **Step 12:** Take out the fragrance oil and place approximately 1/2 teaspoon of each individual oil (1/2 clove, 1/2 thyme, 1/2 cinnamon) inside of the melted wax.
- **Step 13:** Gently stir the fragrance oil in with the melted wax. We use leftover chopsticks because they can be thrown away afterwards.
- **Step 14:** Let the wax harden for 24 hours before lighting it for the first time. After it's hardened, you can cut the excess wick and it's now ready to use.

The mold candles we made are extremely effective. After making them, they were tested with an air quality meter which confirmed the effectiveness.

Quitting Nicotine

As I'm writing this section, the only thing I am thinking of is...nicotine. For 12 years I was addicted to nicotine, whether in the form of chewing tobacco, or nicotine gum. During the addiction, I would typically go through 2 cans of tobacco a day, or 12 pieces of 4mg nicotine infused gum. The addiction proved so strong, that I was unable to function "normally" without a piece of nicotine gum in my mouth. That was until I decided to quit.

Quitting chewing tobacco was easy for me, because I had the nicotine gum to curb my cravings. Quitting the gum though, proved to be a lot harder. For years I grew dependent on nicotine and would rely on it from the moment I woke up until the moment I fell asleep. In my head I firmly believed that chewing the gum was better than using chewing tobacco and therefore justified my usage. The reason for quitting the gum was simple, it was the only variable left in my life that I hadn't experimented with in regards to healing my body. I had tried everything from switching my diet, to avoiding EMFs, and remained at a consistent 90% health status. So, I considered that the final 10% was due to my nicotine use and decided to experiment by not using any for an entire day.

Day 1 results: I ate more than I normally do in a day, possibly because I was trying to keep my mouth busy. Not thinking of nicotine was impossible to do and I ended up cheating and chewing 1 piece of gum.

The fact that I was able to go an entire day on a single piece of gum astonished me but at the same time left me feeling disappointed. I set out that day with the intention of avoiding nicotine all day, and couldn't do it. That is when I created somewhat of a mantra in my head, "if you want to reach 100% health, then you will quit nicotine". Repeating that mantra over and over again was what led me to days 2 and 3 of experimenting with my body's addiction to nicotine.

Day 2 results: I ate even more than I had the previous day and believe it definitely had to do with trying to compensate for the lack of nicotine chewing. I thought of nicotine every second of the day and began singing "nicotine nico nicotine nico" over and over again. I ended the day without using any nicotine but felt strong urges constantly.

Day 3 results: My appetite continued to be larger than normal as I consumed more food than I would in an entire week. My cravings for nicotine increased but my mantra kept me from caving. I truly believed that if I were going to get better then quitting nicotine was the last step. I ended that day without using any nicotine as well.

After day 3, the cravings for nicotine hadn't lessened but the need to maintain a healthy body was more motivating. It has been one of the hardest things I have ever had to do, and I have no intention of ever using nicotine ever again. If I was capable of beating mold illness, Lyme disease and EHS, then beating nicotine will be a walk in the park. That however, is not the truth. The truth is that it is extremely difficult and regardless of the illnesses I have beaten and their individual difficulties, quitting nicotine has proven to be far more difficult than I assumed. That to me is motivating in itself and has helped keep me on the path of resisting nicotine all together.

Earthing

Earthing was one of the worst ideas I ever tried and caused me to feel worse than I had in a long time. From the research I conducted on EHS, numerous studies claimed that Earthing would cure me of my symptoms, and therefore I decided to give it a try. Earthing is basically grounding your body by walking barefoot on the Earth while attempting to connect with the natural energetic resonances of the earth. If walking barefoot on the Earth isn't possible, alternative methods were recommended. I tried both methods, each proving to be more of a danger to my health then a benefit.

My backyard in Arizona was mainly dirt, and had small decorative rocks scattered around as well. For my first attempt at Earthing, I decided to walk outside in my backyard, barefoot. Within seconds of walking barefoot on the dirt and rocks, I felt as if something was working. My toes began to vibrate, then my legs, and eventually my entire body. After a few minutes of thinking that this was going to cure me, my mind quickly shifted to the thought that something bad was happening. I then ran inside, put my socks and shoes back on and noticed that I felt worse than I had in a long time. My body remained in a state of vibration the rest of that night, preventing me from getting any sleep. The next day I decided to test my body voltage while standing in my backyard barefoot. The results were worse than I had thought and revealed that walking barefoot outside allowed over 4,000mV (4 volts) of electricity to enter my body from my bare feet. I assumed at that point that the individuals claiming that Earthing works, were referring to walking in areas where the ground was not electrified and decided to try one of the alternative methods mentioned in the research.

The alternative methods for Earthing was called "grounding". This was achieved by purchasing various grounding products such as pillows or sheets, and plugging them into the ground portion of an outlet and then sleeping on these products. The first product I purchased in order to ground myself was a grounding pillowcase. It was essentially a typical pillowcase but had a metal mesh intertwined inside of it, and a long wire attached to it that was used to plug into my wall. The first night of sleeping with the grounded pillowcase, I felt different but could not put into words what the difference was so I used it for an additional night. That next night I tested my body voltage which of course read 0mV because my body was grounded via the pillowcase. However, my body had more vibrations occurring than I had had while walking outside barefoot.

That night I felt jittery, had extreme vibrations, and couldn't sleep at all. That same feeling followed me into the next day and had me acting as if I had drunk 10 cups of coffee. It wasn't a good feeling to be that hyper and eventually wore off, leaving me feeling sluggish and tired. It was then that I determined that due to excess EMFs in today's world, the grounding pillow I used acted more like an antenna while allowing stray voltage from my environment to enter my body more easily. This was not shown on my body voltage meter because the pillowcase was grounded, therefore completing the circuit upon testing the levels within the body. This was discovered through my ability to feel the effects of the grounding products. The explanation used to explain what was occurring while using these products was as follows:

1. Imagine a large open beach in the middle of the night.
2. In the middle of the sand, imagine a large metal rod with a cable coming off it.
3. Now imagine there being thunder and lighting.
4. Now imagine that you are holding the cable that is attached to the metal rod. Testing your body voltage at this point would be zero because you are grounded through the pole and cable.
5. Now imagine the pole being struck with lightening. That lightening travels into the pole and through the cable, eventually making its way to your body.
6. The pole, while thought of as a grounding device, actually becomes an antenna and attracts the lighting to your body.

Using the above scenario and replacing the lighting for stray electricity in your environment, you are essentially turning your body into an antenna within your home. Maybe if the environment was EMF free, with no power at all, would I give it a try again. That environment does not exist today and therefore I will not be trying grounding again. Earthing on the other hand, is something that I would like to try in an environment that does not have cables running through the ground or stray voltage returning back to the electricity companies. However, finding an environment where that doesn't occur in our modern world has proven to be somewhat of a challenge. I would much rather avoid touching anything that may turn my body into an antenna as the EMF lightening of today bombards our world.

Rebounding

When I first became aware that there was something wrong with my body, I tried figuring it out on my own. One of the conclusions I came to was that my lymphatic system was clogged and therefore it needed to be unclogged or "drained". Figuring that out was mainly just a guess based off of my symptoms, but eventually it proved to be an actual problem. While trying to learn about ways to drain my lymphatic system I came across various drainage methods, but my favorite involved a trampoline.

According to my research, by jumping up and down on a trampoline the lymphatic system gets additional help draining lymphatic fluid, and since you have more lymphatic fluid in your body than you do blood, it seemed rather important. However, it's not called "jumping up and down", its actually referred to as "rebounding". After learning about rebounding I purchased a small trampoline and decided to give it a try. Afterall, who doesn't like jumping on a trampoline?

For the first few days I bounced up and down on the trampoline for 5 minutes a day. Now, 5 minutes may not have seemed like a lot, but when you aren't feeling well it seems like a lot longer. Honestly, I couldn't tell a difference after those few days of rebounding and eventually decided to step up my time bouncing. For an entire week after that I rebounded 15 minutes a day at a minimum and thought that would do the trick. It didn't. Eventually I stopped rebounding because I didn't feel like it was working and because I didn't have access to a trampoline anymore (thrown away during mold remediation). Sometimes now I pretend like I have a trampoline still and jump up and down while pretending I'm still on it. Let me tell you though, it's definitely not the same thing.

Throwing Out Everything

One of the most outrageous things that I had to do when I discovered that I had mold illness, was throw out everything that I owned. Not knowing where the mold originated from meant that I was unsure of what items I owned that had been infested and therefore everything had to go. Everything that I had purchased from clothes to furniture and even old pictures, all had to be thrown out in order to avoid risking re-exposure.

Apparently, this was something that was well known within the community of people suffering from mold illness. If you have mold inside your home, it is a safer idea to get rid of the items infested with it than it is to try and remediate the mold. The doctor that I was seeing had an actual checklist of items she recommended were thrown away in order to be "safe". From what I was told, mold cannot be killed with bleach, that just makes it come back stronger. Mold also grows at an outrageous rate of 600x faster around EMFs. Mold cannot be painted over, washed away, or hidden behind a picture frame (all things that I asked the doctor). If I was going to heal from being exposed to mold then I had to eliminate anything that could potentially have mold on it or that had been exposed.

So, I threw everything that I owned away. That's right, I threw out all of my clothes, books, furniture, jewelry, trophies, awards, shoes, pictures, my bed, and every other thing that I had purchased during my adult life as well as everything I had accrued since I was a child. At that point, everything that I owned was located on my body, which just so happened to be a shirt, sweatshirt, a pair of underwear, socks, shorts, and a pair of shoes. When I left the house where I believe I was exposed to mold, I threw away those clothes and had truly gotten rid of everything from my past. Although that may have been extreme, it was worth it in my opinion. Being sick with mold illness was something that I would never want a chance at being re-exposed to.

To this day, everything that I own fits into three clear tubs. Besides those tubs I also own a single television, a DVD player, a dresser, a bed, and a single night stand. It may seem like a huge sacrifice having to live this way but its only temporary. In the future, once I move to a safe EMF proof environment, ill purchase things that ill actually need. Until then I'm fine wearing the same thing every day, and using plastic utensils. Life is simple.

Chapter 6

Threats to My Recovery

The road to recovery has been one that I have walked predominately alone. It was filled with numerous challenges and obstacles, but with sheer determination I was able to overcome the majority of them. Yet, I am still not at the point where I am able to function fully outside of my home environment and surrounded by EMFs. Unfortunately, the world today is based on technology and is no longer safe for individuals suffering from EHS. Many EHS people have resorted to living off the grid in order to avoid the constant bombardment of EMFs as well as the symptoms that accompany them. For me, there are only a few threats to my recovery that I am concerned about and would prefer not to have to run into the mountains in order to avoid them.

Not having a support system is one of the main threats to my recovery. Having a support system that comforts you, takes care of you, and most of all believes you is crucial. The journey towards health is long, so the more people you have pushing you forward, the better.

Prior to having any resemblance of a support system, I struggled with speaking up. I kept quiet about the pain I was going through on a daily basis. Mainly because whenever I brought up any of my symptoms, I was made to feel crazy. It took meeting a certain woman, to give me my voice again.

Meeting her family for the first time, I expected it to be the same sort of interaction I had been used to with my family. It was the exact opposite with them. They turned off their Wi-Fi, had their phones on airplane mode, and even unplugged their Bluetooth devices before I even arrived. Knowing I was electrically sensitive was enough for them to take the necessary precautions to ensure my comfort while being in their home.

At my family's house, it's a completely different story. Turning off the Wi-Fi was never an option. Asking them to do so resulted in a long list of excuses as to why they needed it to be on. With my own family, I had no voice.

Having my fiancés family as my support system has given me my voice back. However, I wish that I had a larger support system. Besides them, I have no one else to discuss how hard it is dealing with EHS. I can only imagine how hard it would be without my fiancé and her family there for me as if they were my own family.

Besides not having a large support system, loneliness

is another threat to my recovery. The loneliness that comes with an invisible illness is an unfortunate partnership. The simple fact that people refuse to believe you unless they see the symptoms for themselves is just sad. If people only knew the effect it took on our hearts, they may think twice before jumping to conclusions.

The loneliness that I am referring to is not one that can be fixed through physical interactions. It is a loneliness that only someone suffering from an invisible illness could understand. For years it was hammered into me by the people that I once trusted that I was crazy and a drug addict. Both statements were untrue and yet they continued to say otherwise. Not a single person in my life at that time stopped to consider that what I was saying was true and decided to make their own judgements of what was going on with me. When in actuality, all that was "wrong with me" was that I was sick with mold illness, Lyme Disease and EHS. Their words and actions pushed me to the point of retreating into a world of my own, refusing to discuss anything regarding my invisible illnesses with the outside world out of fear of judgement. They made me feel alone with my illness and have continued to do so to this day. Thinking about how alone I felt in those moments sets me back in my recovery. I get fearful that if I discuss my story with anyone that doesn't understand what it's like to be chronically ill with an invisible illness, that I'll be made to feel that loneliness alone.

After going through everything I've been through, there's not a whole lot left in this world that scares me. 5G however, terrifies me to my very core. 5G is the fifth generation of cellular connectivity and will require small cell towers placed on every street corner. The very few times I've been around 5G have been some of the most painful moments I've lived through and its complete activation is a true threat to my recovery.

If everything in this world will soon be interconnected through 5G, then what will that mean for me and the millions of people suffering with EHS? Will we be forced to live our remaining years locked inside our homes? It doesn't seem fair that there truly won't be anywhere for people to go who do not want to be bombarded by extremely high levels of radio frequency radiation. It scares me to think that I may have to live the rest of my life inside in order to avoid these EMFs, alone and without a large support system that understands the pain that I go through being EHS.

Rather than living in fear though, I wrote a book discussing my story as well as all of the weird symptoms and strange things I tried during my journey to health. It is my hope that I will reach others out there that are feeling the loneliness that I have felt, or change the minds of those who are refusing to support someone with an invisible illness. There's not a whole lot that I can do about 5G, but maybe if this book reaches enough people, I will be able to write a new book discussing what others have done to live in a world with 5G.

For those of you who are reading this book and are suffering from an "invisible illness", know that you are not alone. I am here for you. I am here for you just like the authors of the many books I read were there for me. Comforting me with their stories of triumph and success at ridding themselves of their invisible disease.

Chapter 7

Basic Overview of EMFs

Electromagnetic Frequencies (EMF) are invisible waves of energy that are comprised of both Electric Fields and Magnetic Fields. Besides Electric and Magnetic Fields, Radio Frequencies and Dirty Electricity fall under the EMF spectrum. Although invisible, EMFs surround us everywhere we go. From natural sources like the earths geomagnetic field to man-made sources like computers, televisions, and cell towers.

In order to understand EMFs as a whole, I'll first explain them individually:

1. Electric Fields are the voltage from one point to another.
2. Magnetic Fields are created from the electrical current flowing along a metallic path.
3. Radio Frequencies are data packed signals that are transferred through the air from one point to another.

4. Dirty Electricity is created by excess oscillation and spikes of frequencies exceeding 60hz while traveling from one point to another.

Unlike the Magnetic Field which needs an electric current in order to be generated, an Electric Field exists without it. For example, when you plug a lamp into a wall, with it off but still plugged in, an Electric Field exists in/surrounding the lamps cord. Once the lamp is switched on, electrical current flows and a Magnetic Field is created in/surrounding the lamps cord. The stronger the electrical current, the further out the Magnetic Field will extend. The higher the voltage, the stronger the Electrical Field will be.

Radio Frequencies are a little simpler to explain. All wireless technology devices work through invisible frequencies traveling through the air. For example, when you send a text message from your cell phone to another cell phone, think about how it gets there. There are no wires connecting the two cell phones, so how does the text message instantly travel from one place to another? It takes the text message, turns it into a frequency and then travels invisibly through the air, eventually making its way to its intended destination. Imagine explaining that to someone 50 years ago.

Dirty Electricity is a poorly understood part of the EMF spectrum. Working backwards is the best way to explain the subject. For example, when you plug your cell phone into a wall outlet, a steady flow of 60hz electricity is expected to charge the device. However, that's not always the case. What do you think would happen to your phone if it were receiving 10 times the amount of electricity it's designed to handle? Well that's what's happening. The electricity coming through your walls should be a constant frequency but it is not, therefore resulting in "Dirty Electricity". The worst part is that it can be created by your neighbor's home and transferred to your home through the connectivity of power lines. Dirty Electricity is created through the inversion process used with solar panels, CFL and other fluorescent light bulbs, dimmer switches, and any other sources that alternate the flow of electricity.

The main difference between man-made EMFs and EMFs found in nature is that man-made EMFs are "pulsed". Natural EMFs like the earths geomagnetic field are not pulsed. In other words:

Man-made EMFs = Alternating Current (A/C)

Natural EMFs = Direct Current (D/C)

In order to fully understand the difference between pulsed and non-pulsed EMFs, the following is an example that involves your imagination. Do not try the example I am about to give, only visualize it.

Imagine yourself laying on the floor. Now imagine someone gently stepping onto your stomach and standing completely still. Could you handle them standing still on your stomach with the constant pressure of their weight on top of you? Most people say yes (depending on how heavy they are), and for this example to work I'm going to assume you did too. Now imagine that same person standing on your stomach but rather than them standing still, they are jumping up and down repeatedly and at different intervals (sometimes they jump fast, sometimes they jump slow). Could you handle them jumping up and down on your stomach for a prolonged period of time? Eventually they are going to hurt you, or even worse break something. How long do you think you would last in that scenario? A few seconds? Minutes?

The first example of the person standing still represents non pulsed EMFs, while the person jumping on your stomach represents pulsed EMFs. Rather than a steady stream of energy, man-made EMFs are pulsed and are constantly "jumping on our cells". Our bodies can't take the constant pulsing and no matter how strong or healthy you are, eventually damage will occur. The damage is occurring on a cellular level, and therefore we don't see the "person jumping on our stomach" and assume that EMFs are safe. Just because you can't see/feel the damage occurring, doesn't mean it's not happening.

Unfortunately, the public is being misled about the damage that is occurring within our bodies on a cellular level. This wouldn't be the first time though, think about the tobacco industry. There was a time when people thought cigarette smoking was safe. EMFs are the new tobacco and the same strategies used to make the public believe smoking was safe are being implemented.

If someone handed you a bag of 100 M&M's and told you that 3 of them inside the bag would kill you, would you eat them? That is exactly the gamble we are taking today in regards to EMFs. The World Health Organization (WHO) classified cell phones as a "possible carcinogen". Meaning that the EMFs emitted from our cell phones could possibly cause cancer. Yet, most people don't know that. There are even warnings within your phone telling you not place the phone directly on our body. But we still keep them in our pockets and use them up against our ears while making calls. Like how the tobacco industry hid the dangers of smoking from the public, history is repeating itself by hiding the dangers of EMFs.

Safety Standards

Think back to 1996 and the cell phone that you had, if you had one. What did it look like? How often did you use it? What all did you use the phone for?

At that time, the safety standards for cell phones were set, and they haven't changed since. Think about how different your cell phone looks now compared to 1996. Besides the difference in physical appearance, what else is different? The technological advancements have turned the 1996 version of your cell phone into a: computer, GPS, video game device, etc., all fitting into the palm of your hand. Oh, and it makes phone calls too. Yet, the safety standards remain the same.

In 1996 the safety standards were based on a phones ability to heat the bodies tissue. Nothing else. Unfortunately, we now know that cell phones do much more than merely heat the tissue and yet the standards of safety haven't been updated. Why is that? Think about that for a second. As new technology comes out, safety standards should be updated. New technology = new problems. That's a pretty fair assumption in my opinion. Imagine if the company you work for hadn't updated its safety standards since 1996. Would you feel safe working there?

Besides updating the safety standards for cell phones, there should be safety standards set on all EMF emitting devices, yet there aren't. People still use their laptops on their laps, stand next to the microwave when it's on, and use wireless technology devices like Bluetooth throughout their daily lives. All because we are unaware of the dangers it poses to our health due to the lack of sufficient safety standards.

Below I have broken down the most common EMF emitting devices by category as well as the current safety standards (if applicable), and the recommended safe levels.

Radio Frequencies (RF)

1. Anything Bluetooth
2. Ring Doorbell
3. Tablets (iPad, kindle, etc.)
4. Cell phones
5. Wi-Fi
6. Smart Meters (Electric, Gas, Water)
7. Cordless Home Phone (DECT)
8. Microwave Ovens
9. Cell Towers

Magnetic Fields (MF)

1. High Voltage Powerlines
2. Breaker Box

3. Faulty wiring in homes
4. Motors
5. Transformers
6. Solar Panels

Electric Fields (EF)

1. Ungrounded 2-prong electronics
2. Power strips
3. Wiring in homes
4. Stray current on water pipes

Dirty Electricity (DE)

1. Compact Fluorescent Lights (CFL)
2. Fluorescent Lights
3. Chargers
4. Solar Panel Inverters
5. Smart Appliances
6. Dimmer Switches

Radio Frequencies (RF) Safety Standards

According to the FCC, a radio frequency level of 10,000,000 µW/m2 is the highest exposure level allowable. On the contrary, Building Biologists recommend levels far lower for their safety standards at .1 µW/m2. Building Biologists are the leading experts on EMFs and have concluded that the safe levels recommended by the government are far too high. As an EHS individual, I typically tell people that staying below .02 µW/m2 is acceptable for healing, but zero is preferred. If you are capable of staying below .02 µW/m2 within your home, then healing may occur quicker. The problem though is that there really isn't anywhere in our world today where radio frequency levels are that low. Below I have broken down the various safety standards and recommended standards in an easy to read format:

1. 10,000,000 µW/m2 = FCC
2. .1 µW/m2 = Building Biologists
3. .02 µW/m2 = EHS Individuals

Magnetic Field (MF) Safety Standards

The FCC has nothing to do with the Magnetic Field safety standards and therefore the standards are recommended by the IEEE (Institute of Electrical and Electronics Engineers). According to the IEEE, 9,040 mG is the highest exposure level allowable. Interestingly, Building Biologists disagree and state that 1 mG should be the highest safe exposure level. As an EHS individual, I would have to agree with Building Biologists, and recommend that staying below 1 mG allows the body to heal while preventing new damage from occurring. Below I have broken down the various safety standards and recommended standards in an easy to read format:

1. 9,040 mG = IEEE
2. 1 mG = Building Biologists
3. 1 mG = EHS Individuals

Electric Field (EF) Safety Standards

Along with Magnetic Fields, the IEEE also recommends the safety standards for Electric Fields. Their recommended highest safe exposure levels are 10,000 V/m. Building Biologists once again disagree and state their recommended highest safe exposure levels at 1.5 V/m. As an EHS individual, Electric Fields are an area that I strongly discourage avoiding, as it raises your body voltage while not allowing your body to heal. Therefore, I recommend avoiding Electric Fields all together and staying at zero volts per meter. Below I have broken down the various safety standards and recommended standards in an easy to read format:

1. 10,000 V/m = IEEE
2. 1.5 V/m = Building Biologists
3. 0 V/m = EHS Individuals

Dirty Electricity (DE) Safety Standards

The area of Dirty Electricity is far more complicated than the other EMFs listed above, and therefore a safety standard hasn't been enforced. According to the creators of the Dirty Electricity Filters, below 25 mV is recommended. Besides that recommendation, I wasn't able to find any governing body that stated safe recommendations. However, being an EHS individual, I can assure you that just like all of the other EMFs, keeping as close to zero as possible is recommended. Below I have broken down the two recommended safety standards in an easy to read format:

1. 25 mV = GreenWave Company
2. 0 mV = EHS Individuals

Meters I Use

Something nobody told me while first discovering the

dangers of EMFs, was that the meters you use matter. There are some meters on the market that are cheap and somewhat reliable, but for people with EHS "somewhat reliable" isn't good enough. The meters I use are expensive, but they are top of the line and the absolute best for detecting EMFs.

At first, I purchased numerous meters that claimed to be the absolute best at detecting EMFs, but eventually I figured out that the meters you use need to be specific. There is no cheap option for detecting the precise levels of EMFs, however there are some cheap options that can tell you if you have a problem or not. Below I will list out the various meters that I use today, as well as the body voltage meter that I invented/patented.

Radio Frequency Field Measurement:

1. HF35C RF Meter (800 MHz-2.5 GHz)
    a. This meter measures a wide range of radio frequencies and was less than 500 dollars. It only measures radio frequencies. One of my favorite things about this device is that it has an audible function on it that allows you to hear what the radio frequencies sound like. Smart meters sound different than Wi-Fi, etc. The reason why I went with this meter rather than the more advanced options is because there is a little screw that you can purchase, that screws onto the antenna area of this meter allowing the range of frequencies to be extended. Essentially

making it the same effectiveness as the more expensive versions. If I were to choose one meter to purchase out of all the meters I own, it would be a radio frequency meter. You would be surprised at how many devices inside and outside your home put off radio frequencies. Plus, the sound scares people.

Electric/ Magnetic Field Measurement:

1. NFA1000 EMF Meter (5 Hz-1,000,000 Hz)
    a. This meter was a couple thousand dollars, but it was well worth the investment. I have tested it against numerous other Electric and Magnetic field meters and this one is the best by far. It is extremely accurate, and also has an audible option so that you can hear the Electric and Magnetic Fields. To be honest with you though, I have found that I use this meter far less than my radio frequency meter, and therefore would only recommend purchasing this if you are going to be doing home inspections. Otherwise, I would invest my money in a radio frequency meter.

Dirty Electricity Measurement:

1. GreenWave Broadband EMI Meter (1-1,900 mVAC)
    a. Besides the Radio Frequency meter,

having a Dirty Electricity meter is also a must have. This meter is extremely easy to use and lets you know just how much of a problem Dirty Electricity is within your home. It was less than 200 dollars and doesn't require any batteries or charging. You simply plug it into an outlet that has power and it works.

Body Voltage Measurement:

1. The Body Voltage Meter
    a. This is a device that I personally developed due to the fact that there wasn't one on the market. It was designed to measure AC electric fields by using your body. Your body voltage is simply just the amount of electricity that is currently going through your body. It should be zero, but you would be surprised at how many people are sleeping in an environment where they have thousands of millivolts of electricity surging through their bodies all night. Due to COVID-19, production on The Body Voltage Meter has been delayed but hopefully soon it will be available in stores. Besides the Radio Frequency meter, and the Dirty Electricity meter, I would recommend purchasing a Body Voltage meter because knowing how much electricity is going through your body at any given time is

important during the process of healing. If you have more than 100mV of electricity surging through your body at any given time, the healing process is halted.

As you can see, there are numerous meters that I use in order to properly detect every area of EMFs. Summing up the ones that I feel are the most important and would be the main ones I would purchase if just now starting out would be:

1. Radio Frequency: HF35C RF Meter
2. Dirty Electricity: GreenWave Broadband EMI
3. Body Voltage Meter

Home Inspection Questionnaire

In order to gain an accurate representation of your current EMF use, whether intentional or unintentional, please fill out the below questionnaire to the best of your ability.

Exterior of House

1. Are there any above ground power lines near your property?
2. Do you have a smart meter? (I.e. gas, electric, water)
3. Can you see a cell tower from anywhere on your property?
4. Do you have solar panels?
5. Are your neighbors' homes close enough to pick up their Wi-Fi?
6. Do you have a wireless security/doorbell

system?
7. Do you have any exterior Bluetooth enabled devices? (i.e. pool lighting, anything that can be controlled by an app on your phone)

Interior of House

1. Do you have Wi-Fi?
2. Do you have a range extender for your Wi-Fi?
3. Do you have a cordless home phone?
4. Do you have a voice automated assistant? (i.e. Alexa, Google assistant)
5. Do you turn your cell phone on "airplane mode" when not in use?
6. Do you have a tablet(s)? (i.e. iPad, kindle)
7. Do you have a "smart tv"?
8. Do you have Bluetooth enabled devices? (i.e. stereo/speakers, headphones, keyboard, mouse, printer, rumba vacuum, tile)
9. Do you have a laptop or home computer?
10. Do you have dimmer switches?
11. Do you leave your electronic appliances plugged in when not in use?
12. Do you use a microwave oven?
13. Do you have an electric stove?
14. Do you have fluorescent/halogen light bulbs?
15. Do you use a hair dryer?
16. Do you use an electric razor or electric toothbrush?
17. Do you have "smart appliances"?
18. Do you sleep near a plugged-in lamp?
19. Do you have a plugged-in alarm clock near where you sleep?
20. Has there ever been mold damage in your home?

21. Do you have a Wi-Fi enabled thermostat? (i.e. Nest)
22. Do you use an electric blanket or electric heating pad?
23. Do you have "smart plugs"?
24. Do you have a Wi-Fi or Bluetooth enabled baby monitor?
25. Do you have a Bluetooth enabled air purifier? (i.e. Molekule)
26. Do you have any video game consoles? (i.e. Xbox, Wii, Nintendo switch, PlayStation)
27. Do you have two or more stories in your home?

Personal

1. Do you carry your cell phone on your body?
2. Do you use speakerphone while talking on your cell phone?
3. Do you wear any "smart" devices? (i.e. Apple Watch, fitness tracker, Fitbit)
4. Do you use Bluetooth enabled headphones?
5. Do you have metal fillings?
6. Do you use metal framed glasses?
7. Do you have any metal in your body? (i.e. metal rod, screws)
8. Do you carry any keyless entry devices on your body? (i.e. car keys)
9. Do you wear a wireless diabetes monitor?
10. Do you have a "smart" or electric car?
11. Do you have Wi-Fi capabilities in your car?
12. Are you using your TV, cell phone, computer or tablet within an hour of falling asleep?

Fill in the blank

1. How many hours a day do you watch television?
2. How many hours a day do you use your cell phone?
3. How many hours a day do you use your computer?
4. How many hours a day do you use your tablet? (i.e. iPad, kindle)
5. How many hours of sleep are you getting per night?
6. Do you have difficulty staying or falling asleep?
7. How long does it take for you to fall asleep?
8. Do you know your body voltage in bed?
9. How many people live in your home?
10. Where is your phone and/or tablet when you are sleeping?
11. How often do you check your cell phone throughout the night?
12. When was the last time you had a home EMF inspection?
13. How many years have you been using a cell phone?
14. How many waking hours per day are you spending technology free?

The intention of the above checklist is to get you thinking of all the EMFs that are currently in your life. Although the list is not fully inclusive, as I do not know your specific situation, it does cover a very large spectrum of average EMF exposure. If you're interested in what follows the home inspection questionnaire please visit: EHSwarrior.com for further details regarding remediation.

Chapter 8

Supplements List

1. **Designs for Health Twice Daily Essential Packets (multivitamin, fish oil, magnesium, calcium)**
    a. Foundational nutrients to support basic chemical reactions in the body and fish oil to decrease inflammation. These packets also contain the niacin needed to assist in NAD+ production. As these come in premade packages, they are easy to travel with and increase compliance.
2. **Bio-Botanical Research Inc. Olivirex**
    a. A high potency olive leaf herbal combination to support the immune system. Olive Leaf is said to help protect against wireless radiation.
3. **Pure Encapsulations Liposomal Glutathione**
    a. Glutathione is a powerful antioxidant and helps support the body in detoxification.

4. **Quicksilver Scientific H2 Elite**
   a. Molecular hydrogen helps increase Nrf2 in the body.
5. **Tru Niagin Pro 500**
   a. Contains nicotinamide riboside chloride, a NAD+ precursor, which helps repair EMF induced DNA damage
6. **Biotics Research Acti-Mag Plus**
   a. A powdered magnesium with B vitamins. Among many of the beneficial benefits of magnesium, it is great for EMF induced damage as it acts as a natural calcium channel blocker.
7. **Biotics Research CoQ-Zyme 30**
   a. CoQ10 is a great antioxidant and important cofactor in the DNA repair PARP pathway. It also helps with muscle pain.
8. **Allergy Research Group Nrf2 Renew**
   a. An antioxidant blend capable of increasing Nrf2 in the body to decrease inflammation.
9. **Klaire Labs Ther-Biotic Complete**
   a. A probiotic containing 25 Billion CFU Multispecies that are good for overall gut health

Chapter 9

Further Reading

Below is a list of some of the physical books I read while healing from Mold, Lyme, and EHS, in regards to EMFs. They are in order of my personal favorites. All of these books were read in paperback versions, rather than online. Although these were not all of the books I read, they were among my favorites.

1. The Invisible Rainbow
    a. By Arthur Firstenburg
2. Zapped
    a. By Ann Louise Gittleman
3. EMF*D
    a. By Dr. Joseph Mercola
4. EMF Freedom
    a. By Elizabeth Plourde, PhD
    b. By Marcus Plourde, PhD
5. Exposed
    a. By Bill Cadwallader
6. The Non-Tinfoil Guide to EMFs
    a. By Nicolas Pineault

7. EMF Practical Guide
    a. By Lloyd Burrell
8. Dirty Electricity
    a. By Samuel Milham, MD, MPH
9. Radiation Nation
    a. By Daniel T. Debaun
    b. By Ryan P. Debaun
10. Toxic
    a. By Neil Nathan, MD
11. Healing Severe Chemical and EMF Sensitivity
    a. By Gary Patera
12. Curing Electromagnetic Hypersensitivity
    a. By Steven Magee
13. Cancer and EMF Radiation
    a. By Brandon LaGreca, Lac, MAcOM
14. Electromagnetic Radiation Survival Guide
    a. By Dr. Jonathan Halpern, PhD

Acknowledgements

Thank you to the Noronha family for feeding me, talking to me, believing in me, being part of my support system, turning off all of your EMFs whenever I was around, and most of all for allowing me to marry your daughter.

Thank you to John at Ketamine for treating me like a person and for taking an actual interest in my condition. You and your company are top notch in my book, literally.

Contact the Author

After writing this book, I have given up the use of a cellphone completely. Which means that contacting me is a little more difficult than before. In order to get ahold of me, please use one of the methods below and I will do my best to get back to you.

Email: Brian@EHSwarrior.com

Website: EHSwarrior.com

Other Books by the Author

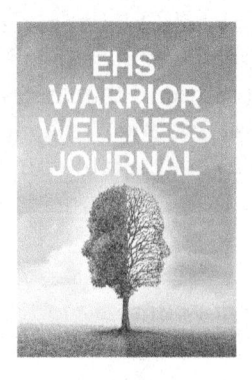

EHS Warrior Wellness Journal

Being electrically sensitive is not fun. There are numerous challenges that we face on a daily basis that a majority of society has no clue about, and it leaves us questioning a lot. This wellness journal was designed with you in mind. Now you will have a place to track your symptoms, track your diet and water intake, track your screen time, schedule your appointments, and provide you with an opportunity to track your progress as you head down your journey towards recover.

Being EHS is difficult, I know that first hand, but it is not impossible to heal from. Why is this important to track? Being EHS it's easy to forget the things that you do on a daily basis to help you get healthy. This wellness journal is the culmination of tracking that I did during my own journey to health and wellness. It is designed specifically for someone with EHS looking to keep track of everything in one place as well as provide an opportunity to look back at the symptoms that you overcame.

This is a 4-month wellness journal, with a full calendar, weekly schedule, daily break down and space for journaling, as well as a weekly symptom tracker with actual EHS symptoms.

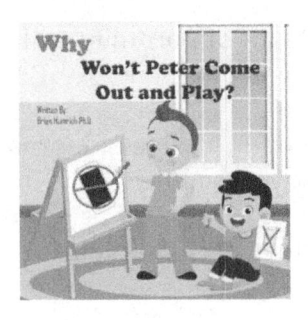

Children's book: Why Wont Peter Come Out and Play?

Cell phones are addicting, at what age should we allow our children to take part in this addiction? The average age for owning a cell phone is now 10 years old. Is that something that you are okay with as a parent? Or would you rather see your child running around and playing outside? I know my answer, but it's up to you to decide if your child will stay inside on the phone all day or go outside and play.

This book is designed for children of all ages and encourages them to choose a childhood free of the distractions a cell phone may impose. Will Peter come out and play? Or will he sit inside on his phone all day? Read this book and find out today!

BRIAN R. HUMRICH

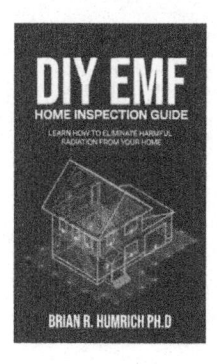

DIY EMF Home Inspection Guide: Learn How to Eliminate Harmful Radiation from your Home

With the recent release of 5G and the ever-expanding field of new technology, finding an environment free of radiation is becoming more and more impossible. Within this guide you will learn step by step how to reduce the harmful radiation in your home through conducting an EMF home inspection. Take control of the EMF radiation in your life and feel the difference immediately by learning how to detect and remediate high sources of radiation from: radio frequencies, magnetic fields, electric fields, and dirty electricity.

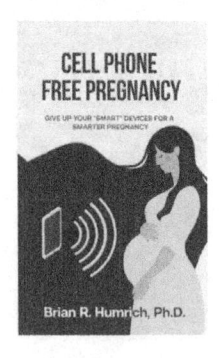

Cell Phone Free Pregnancy: Give up your "smart" devices for a smarter pregnancy

Did you know that your cell phone emits radio frequency radiation that is twice as dangerous to an infant than an adult? Or that the radiation emitted from your wifi router can cause learning disabilities in your child? Join the movement sweeping the nation of mothers-to-be putting down their cell phones, turning off their wifi routers, and getting rid of their "smart" devices. The goal is a healthier pregnancy, the results are much more than that. In this book you will learn why a cell phone free pregnancy is a smarter pregnancy, as well as tips and tricks on how to eliminate harmful radiation from your life. The science is there and the results are clear, cell phones are out and healthy pregnancies are in.

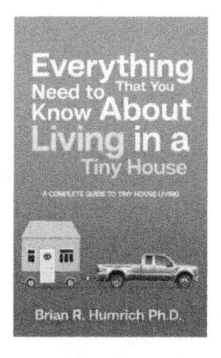

Everything That You Need to Know About Living in a Tiny House: A Complete Guide to Tiny House Living

Find out if the tiny house lifestyle is for you in this captivating book about all of the ins and outs people won't tell you about tiny house living. Learn about everything from securing a mortgage, to what it's like having zero privacy, and even how to change a flat tire. If you are considering tiny house living and don't know where to start, start here.

EHS WARRIOR